community mental health programs in england

community mental health programs in england

AN AMERICAN VIEW

by
Norman Rosenzweig, M.D.

SINAI HOSPITAL OF DETROIT
WAYNE STATE UNIVERSITY

with a foreword by Howard P. Rome, M.D.

WAYNE STATE UNIVERSITY PRESS DETROIT, 1975

*Published simultaneously in Canada
by the Copp Clark Publishing Company
517 Wellington Street, West
Toronto 2B, Canada.*

Library of Congress Cataloging in Publication Data

*Rosenzweig, Norman, 1924-
Community mental health programs in England.*

*Bibliography: p.
1. Community mental health services–Great
Britain. I. Title. [DNLM 1. Community mental
health services–England. WM30 R816c]
RA790.7.G7R67 1974 362.2'2'0942 74-13365
ISBN 0-8143-1524-0*

To
Carol
and
Betty Ann

contents

illustrations

maps and charts

Maps and Charts

foreword

Our British colleagues, as Dr. Norman Rosenzweig has observed, have been most innovative in creating, then periodically modifying their health-care delivery system since the termination of World War II. The advent of socialized medicine brought the government as an official third party into the doctor-patient relationship which previously had been held to be a sacrosanct dual relationship. Then too, for a complex of reasons, this action permitted experimentation with a variety of alternate therapeutic techniques on an institution-wide scale. In turn, this gave rise to a number of adjunctive facilities for the care and management of mentally ill patients.

The pioneer studies conducted at Belmont Hospital, Epsom Downs, by Dr. Maxwell Jones initiated the concept of a "therapeutic community." Jones noted, "It is the introduction of trained staff personnel into the group situation together with planned collaboration of patients and staff in most, if not all, aspects of the unit life which heightens the possibility of the social experience being therapeutic" (Jones, Maxwell. 1953. "The Therapeutic Community: A New Treatment Method in Psychiatry," New York: Basic Books).

In Great Britain, the term "social psychiatry" refers to intramural or extramural therapeutic communities. With medical care being accepted as an individual right as well as a public good, everyone has an equal opportunity to admittance to basic facilities and to be offered services of a generally acceptable standard. This is the aim of the National Health Service: to provide effective psychiatric service to the patient, his family, and the community. An important dimension in the entire plan is the conviction that prompt early treatment during the crisis episode will preclude admission to mental hospitals with its expensive and personally dislocating effects. A corollary is the creation of special outpatient resources to care for the special needs of psychiatric patients.

The context within which these psychiatric services must be seen is an historic one. Public mental hospitals, or county lunatic asylums as they were known, had been built under a permissive act of 1808. They developed rapidly in the second half of the 19th century. A society of asylum doctors became the Royal Medico-Psychological Association in 1841; it became the major spokesman for psychiatry. At the time of World War I and thereafter, there was an affiliation of specialists (consultants) with one or the other of the Royal Colleges of Medicine or Surgery. Psychiatry advanced in its status with the creation by the Conjoint Board of a Diploma in Psychological Medicine (DPM) in 1920. The majority of psychiatrists continued outside of the mainstream of general medicine, which was represented by the Royal College of Physicians in which the membership issue of a separate college for psychiatrists was debated until 1964. Part of the reason was the disadvantaged position that psychiatry held in medical education. For example, in 1938, there were only nine psychiatric beds in the London undergraduate teaching hospitals, of a total bed complement of 6,700.

There also was a dichotomy in the character of staffing of the hospitals; the large voluntary hospitals were staffed by specialists-consultants and were intimately associated with medical teaching, whereas the smaller voluntary hospitals were staffed by general practitioners who also performed what specialty services were required.

Then too, there was the progressively widening gap between the generalist and the specialist in Britain during these years. This too was reflected in the quality of service being provided by the relatively disorganized voluntary hospital system until the creation in 1948 under the National Health Service of the present regionalized hospital service. It brought into sharp focus the need for standards and their creation as well as the ensuing controversy in which the British Medical Association was heavily involved as to who of its members was to do what and where. Some 11,000 specialists and other medical practitioners were working in hospitals, and some 18,000 general medical practitioners entered the National Health Service on July 5, 1948.

Psychiatry as a specialty accounted for 2.3 per cent of the specialists in 1938-39; by 1964 the percentage of psychiatrists had reached 10 per cent. The rapid expansion of sub-specialty knowledge and technique posed a problem for the Royal College of Physicians. Professor D. K. Henderson, president of the Royal Medico-Psychological Association in 1946 said, "Psychiatry is the other half of medicine and just not another specialty." He expressed the syncretic point of view. It was not until the

1960s that psychiatry became organizationally distinct from its parent organizational body, internal medicine.

It needs to be pointed out that specialization in Britain as well as in the United States has engendered a crisis in undergraduate and postgraduate medical education which also is reflected in the facilities in which the specialty is practiced. These issues are by no means settled today. There has been a waxing proliferation of related subspecialties (e.g., child psychiatry, forensic psychiatry, subnormality, etc.) and special techniques designed to cope with their unique problems. These have led to the creation of special settings in which these functions can be best performed.

British psychiatry has undergone many significant changes in recent times in its professional organizational structure, with the conversion of the Royal Medico-Psychological Association to the Royal College of Psychiatrists. Everything from its examination and accreditation procedures to an individual recognition as a Royal College are accouterments of psychiatry's enhanced status. Dr. Rosenzweig's survey of these salient features, especially as they reflect the viewpoint of an experienced American psychiatrist-educator-administrator, brings into focus a much-needed critical perspective of the problems confronted, involved, and yet to be resolved. He portrays a mental-health delivery system which can be compared and contrasted with our own mental health center system.

Howard P. Rome, M.D.
Consultant, Mayo Clinic
Rochester, Minnesota

President, World Psychiatric Association

preface

The purpose of this book is to acquaint the American health care professional with a system of mental health care that is significantly different from his own. It is based on a study made during a three-month sabbatical spent as a visiting scientist at the Tavistock Institute, London, in 1969, followed by a second visit in 1971, and it represents a transcultural study of community mental health services in England. Initially, I intended to discover what contributions the British had made to the methodology of community mental health, since many of the innovations introduced into the United States were traceable to earlier programs in England. I also wished to ascertain what type of progress had been made within the British system, what kinds of approaches had succeeded and what kinds had failed.

The situation that I encountered forced me to alter my original intentions. First, there is a marked cultural disparity between England and the United States which is not immediately apparent because of the superficial similarity of language and the assumption that we mean the same things when we use the same words. In addition, the developmental background, social organization, relationships between individuals both professional and nonprofessional, and the overall outlook of the two countries differ in important ways. Social institutions, although they may bear the same name in the two countries, do not represent the same things; in fact, what is meant by community mental health in England is not the same as what is meant by community mental health in the United States. To understand the British system of mental health care, it is first necessary to become acquainted with the context of the British system and the ways in which it differs from the context of health services in the United States.

A second distinction is immediately apparent. In the British system of "socialized medicine," mental health care and other health services are obtained through the National Health Service, free of charge to everyone. In the United States, mental health and other health services are obtained chiefly through a system oriented toward private practice. This fact in itself indicates a level of acceptance of psychiatric services by the general public or at least by the middle class, who make up the bulk of the population. The average consumer of psychiatric services in the United States expects to be evaluated and treated with some degree of regularity over a prolonged period of time, often with the intention of altering his underlying psychic structure. A system of mental health care oriented toward private practice did not gain a significant foothold in England because of the way that health care in general has evolved since the Middle Ages. Within the structure of "socialized medicine" instituted after World War II there was no place for it.

In Britain the neurotic person is often accepted as just another member of the community, because there is an unusually high tolerance for eccentricity. The British do not usually seek psychiatric assistance unless there is some danger of suicide or homicide or some kind of irrational behavior that makes a person completely unmanageable at home. The goal of the health service is to bring the disturbing symptoms under control and, if possible, to maintain the patient either at home or in some kind of community setting, such as a hostel or sheltered workshop. Community organizations help individuals to deal with problems related to housing, education, or government red tape, but more as a means of helping citizens to cope with socialistic governmental functions than as a mental health service. Efforts such as those of St. Christopher's Hospice in dealing with the problems of death, dying, and the bereaved, and voluntary agencies such as the Citizens' Advice Bureaux and the Council of Social Services all provide services which in the United States would be considered as related to mental health but which are not so considered in England.

The two countries differ also in the very nature of the social changes that they have undergone. I conceptualize change as being of two kinds: unplanned change, that is, evolution or process in either a growing or deteriorating direction; and planned or revolutionary change, brought about through the direct intervention of man for a particular purpose or goal. Both forms of change have an impact, but the first comes about as a consequence of forces acting without a particular goal; the outcome is a consequence of interacting forces, natural and non-natural, over time. It may occur without anyone's awareness that it is taking place. With goal-directed change, some decision is made as to what the final outcome should be and circumstances are manipulated accordingly. Not infrequently, a particular vested interest is promoted at the expense of other interests. Planned change is rapid and tends to shake up the system. Generally, it meets considerable resistance because it upsets the status quo; life patterns are more suddenly disrupted and new relationships have to be established over a short period of time.

At the time of my first visit to the Tavistock Centre in 1969, community mental health programs in England had developed almost entirely through unplanned change. From a point in 1948, when the National Health Service took over the mental hospitals, events seemed to follow as natural evolutionary consequences. The hospitals became overcrowded and individual attempts were made to solve this problem. Tranquilizers made it possible to move some patients from institutional to community facilities; workshops were established in the hospitals to give industrial training; and community agencies and the local authorities (local governments in England) were encouraged to create centers, such as hostels, to handle patients in the community. Subsequent legislative changes prior to 1971 were usually intended to consolidate the evolutionary gains. These legislative enactments served to disseminate information about those innovations found to be satisfactory solutions to local problems, so that others might emulate them.

In the United States, however, the community mental health program came about as a planned change. The findings and recommendations of the Presidential Commission appointed by President Dwight D. Eisenhower in 1958, which were reported in the book *Action for Mental Health,* led to the community mental health legislation of 1963 (16), one of the last bills signed by President John F. Kennedy before his assassination. Among other requirements, this legislation called for the construction of community mental health centers with certain characteristics mandated by Washington.

By the time of my 1971 visit, mental health care and other aspects of the British postwar socialized medicine had been found inadequate to the needs of consumers, and many studies were consequently in progress to remedy the inadequacies. A Royal Commission, appointed to reorganize the patterns of local government, was proposing to change the geographic boundaries and to modify the relationships of the smaller units of the local government to the larger central government (58). Other commissions were re-evaluating the education of health care professionals, particularly physicians and social workers.

The role of social services (in a country that had adopted socialism) had been investigated by the Seebohm Committee in 1968 (101). At that time the social work staff (psychiatric social workers) of the mental health sections of the local authority health departments were the real providers of community mental health services. The implementation of the

Seebohm Report (Report of the Committee on Local Authority and Allied Personal Social Services) in 1971, established a separate local authority Social Service Department. Thereafter psychiatric social workers were grouped with social workers from the Children's Department and the Welfare Department, all of whom assumed the role of generic social workers.

The implementation of the Seebohm Report was one instance of revolutionary change that I encountered on my return to England. It required that I modify my original assessments and descriptions of many programs. I revisited a number of places and engaged in discussions and correspondence with many people to understand the full implications of the changes. Some of the disruptions I noted were undoubtedly superficial, resulting from the reorganization necessary when relationships are shifted, and from the consequent resistance to reorganization. Other disruptions, more deeply rooted, would undoubtedly have far-reaching consequences. It was difficult to distinguish among them.

In addition to describing the hospitals and programs that I observed, I have discussed the administrative modifications during both the pre-Seebohm and post-Seebohm stages of community mental health care; the Redcliffe-Maud Report (58) concerning local government reorganization; the unification of the health services recommended in the Second Green Paper (40), in the Tripartite Committee Report (45), and finally, in the White Paper (59); the Health Ministry's proposal to develop psychiatric units in district general hospitals (42); modifications in the medical school curriculum (57); the formation of the new Royal College of Psychiatrists (67); and some of the reports issued by the Society of Clinical Psychiatrists on subjects ranging from administration to architecture to care of children and old people (23, 68, 78, 100). Since many proposals will be implemented in 1974, changes will deluge the community, possibly at the time this volume is due to appear. I have tried to assess the implications and potential consequences of these planned changes.

I have divided the book into two parts. Part I deals with the background and the context of mental health services, the service elements, and the ways in which they differ from those familiar to most Americans. It is organized in a way which I felt might help the reader to understand the overall contrast between British and American systems of mental health care and social organization. Part II consists of specific descriptions of particular programs and hospitals which illustrate the concepts developed in Part I. In addition, I have included a discussion of the community mental health and related services available to a particular borough of London.

My observations are drawn, for the most part, from places of good reputation suggested to me as providing examples of particular types of programs. I have not attempted a comprehensive survey, nor are any of the programs "typical." To keep the scope of my book within reasonable bounds, I did not describe all the places that I visited. Omissions should not be construed as reflection upon the quality of any program.

I am indebted to many people for help in identifying and visiting programs, as well as in collecting the data. I am particularly indebted to Dr. Joshua Bierer and Dr. C. Murray Parkes, both of whom were largely instrumental in calling my attention to programs and helping to make arrangements for my visits.

Beyond this, I am especially grateful to Dr. John Howells, who has kept me abreast of developments by means of personal reports, by forwarding to me relevant articles from the press and scientific journals, and for seeing to it that I received all relevant official publications as they appeared.

At each of the places I visited, many people gave patiently of their time and assistance, guiding me through, describing programs and directing me to additional information. I am thankful for the generosity and hospitality of them all.

The list of those to whom I am indebted would itself fill a chapter. However, I would like to make special acknowledgement of the aid rendered to me by the following people: Dr. Bernard Adams, Dr. Maurice Baird, Dr. Douglas Bennett, Dr. James Birley, Dr. John Bowlby, Dr. Felix Brown, Dr. Norman Capstick, Dr. M. S. DeMowbray, Dr. F. R. Dennison, Dr. J. D. W. Fisher, Dr. Hugh Freeman, Mr. and Mrs. Ford, Dr. Richard Gosling, Mrs. Anthea Hailey, Dr. Wilfred Harding, Mrs. Martha Harris, Dr. Dorothy Heard, Dr. R. A. Hobdell, Dr. H. M. Holden, Dr. W. L. Jones, Dr. J. H. Kahn, Dr. Marion MacKenzie, Dr. B. M. Mandelbrote, Mrs. R. M. Marre, Miss A. Murphy, Miss P. M. Perrott, Dr. Peter Sainsbury, Dr. Cicely Saunders, Dr. Maurice Silverman, Dr. R. Wilkins, and Drs. John and Lorna Wing.

I wish also to express my appreciation to Dr. Hilda Griscom for her editorial assistance, and to Miss Barbara Grembos, Mrs. Alice Freeman Smith, Mrs. Betty Taylor, and Miss Christine Williamson for their secretarial efforts.

PART ONE: THE BACKGROUND

Abbreviations and Terms

AHA	Area Health Authority
AHA(T)	Teaching Area Health Authority
CAB	Citizens' Advice Bureaux
DRO	Disablement Resettlement Officer
DPM	Diploma in Psychological Medicine
DUIT	Day Unit for Industrial Therapy (Mapperley Hospital)
FPC	Family Practitioner Committee
IMS	Institute of Marital Studies (Tavistock Centre)
IRU	Industrial Rehabilitation Unit
ITU	Industrial Therapy Unit
MACA	Mental After-Care Association
MOH	Medical Officer of Health
MRC	Medical Research Council
MWO	Mental Welfare Officer
PSW	Psychiatric Social Worker
RHA	Regional Health Authority
RCPsych	Royal College of Psychiatrists
RMN	Registered Mental Nurse
RMPA	Royal Medico-Psychological Association
RNMS	Registered Nurse for the Mentally Subnormal
RSCN	Registered Sick Children's Nurse
SEN	State Enrolled Nurse
SRN	State Registered Nurse
YPCS	Young Peoples Counselling Service (Tavistock Centre)

1

Some comparisons of the community mental health programs in Britain and the United States

Many elements of the community mental health programs of the United States have been derived from innovations developed in Britain. These include such approaches as the open-door policy, the therapeutic community, the use of day hospitals and partial hospitalization, therapeutic social clubs, and industrial therapy workshops. Furthermore, the implementation of a community mental health program under national auspices occurred in Britain five years before such a program was inaugurated in the United States. It should therefore be of interest to Americans involved in planning and implementing community programs to examine the developments in Britain since the inception of their mental health program in 1959.

For an American to understand the British program, it is first necessary to appreciate the significant differences in the political and social organizations between the two countries, for these factors have a major relevance for the shaping of community programs. In Britain responsibility for providing services is divided between the Health Department of the central government and the Public Health Authority of the local government (called the local authority). The Health Department operates the mental hospitals and employs the psychiatric specialists. The Public Health Authority is responsible, by statute, for providing services for the mentally retarded and mentally ill, including admissions to hospitals and aftercare following discharge, particularly through community-based programs. Thus, while the American program emphasizes comprehensiveness and continuity of care, the division of responsibilities in England makes such comprehensiveness and continuity difficult to achieve. Successful programs in England have in fact been those created by ingenious individuals who have devised schemes for bridging the gap between local authority and Health Ministry services. Each such ingenious scheme is, therefore, unique and not characteristic of community mental health systems as a whole.

Another major distinction between the health services of the two countries is that practically all doctors in Britain are employed by the National Health Service, while in the United States most physicians are in private practice. In Britain almost everyone wishing to avail himself of medical services must make use of those services provided by the National Health scheme. In the United States, particularly with the widespread availability of health insurance, most middle-income people are accustomed to approaching health services privately. Only the lower-income groups have been more accustomed to obtain these services from clinics or other institutional providers. Since the latter group is the one which has tended in the past to utilize mental health services least, there has resulted a dual pattern of utilization of mental health services in the United States; the middle class have tended to see psychiatrists privately for much milder disorders, such treatment even having in some areas a positive status value; while on the other hand, the lower socio-economic groups have been inclined to utilize psychiatric services only for severe illnesses which cannot be coped with other than by institutionalization. The task of developing community mental health services in the United States, therefore, involves both a reorganization of middle-class patterns of seeking psychiatric services, as well as an attempt to reach and educate the lower socio-economic groups to the importance of seeking psychiatric assistance much earlier in the course of events and to the availability of services providing earlier treatment.

In Britain, treatment of mild neuroses by psychotherapy is comparatively rare. Such treatment is not readily available within the Health Service, because there are too few psychiatrists and too many patients with major disorders for a doctor to give much attention to the minor problems and especially to set aside the blocks of time required for psychotherapeutic sessions; and also because most British psychiatrists are poorly trained in dynamic psychiatry and tend to be antagonistic to Freudian ideas. Thus, the handful who would seek such treatment must obtain it at personal expense from a small minority who practice psychoanalysis or dynamic psychotherapy privately. The bulk of the population have tended to steer clear of psychiatry except when they could not avoid doing so, and the pattern of utilization of mental health services has been for the majority of Britons, regardless of class, similar to the pattern characteristic for blue-collar Americans. Psychiatrists and psychiatric services have been centered in hospitals, and the task of the community mental health program in Britain has been essentially to shift this focus from the institution to community-based facilities. It does not require a major reorganization of patterns of utilization such as the situation in the United States would require, although it certainly has involved an education of the public aimed at gaining community acceptance of the mental patient and reducing the stigma of mental illness. The success of this educational effort was attested by the results of a public opinion poll, published in the *Sunday Times,* October 17, 1971, which reported "strong public support for integrating the mentally ill into the community rather than confining them in institutions."

There are also differences between American and British psychiatrists in professional background, training, and orientation, which are reflected in their respective attitudes towards and interpretations of community psychiatry. The widespread influence of psychoanalytic concepts in American psychiatry has led many practitioners to focus their interest and attention upon the inner psychodynamics of the individual patient, particularly those forces considered responsible for the genesis of his illness. The American psychiatrist is thus often suspicious of approaches which shift the focus away from the individual. Even when he does interest himself in social factors, he tends to retain his genetic orientation; that is, he concentrates upon the extra-individual forces in the community which have impinged upon the personality and which are considered to contribute to the development of mental illness. For such a psychiatrist, community psychiatry represents a concern with epidemiology and prevention of emotional disorder.

Most British psychiatrists work in mental hospitals, where they must spread their efforts thinly among great numbers of patients. They could not become deeply involved with individual personality dynamics even if they were so inclined and trained, and most are neither. They tend to be organically oriented, to view their patients in physical terms, and to focus upon nosology, overt symptomatology, and functional disability. They can therefore accept more readily than their American counterparts the notion of dealing with populations rather than individuals, and tend to view community psychiatry as being concerned with reduction of symptoms, retraining of functional capacities, and social reintegration into community life—in other words, rehabilitation.

As a consequence, community mental health programs in the two countries have had differences in emphasis. In the United States, the focus has been upon preventive aspects. Community centers for reaching disadvantaged groups have been developed to provide help in coping with problems of living, since such coping failures are considered to contribute to the development of disabling psychiatric illness. Emphasis has also been placed on early case finding and crisis intervention. In Britain, emphasis has been placed at the other end of the system. Programs have been directed at mobilization of chronically ill patients from custodial institutions into the community, with a considerable stress on social and industrial rehabilitation and the provision of hostels, half-way houses, and other sheltered living and work facilities in the community.

This is not to say that over time the two approaches have not moved closer together. In the United States there has been in recent years increasing emphasis upon efforts to reduce state hospital populations, not only through finding alternatives to admission in the first place, but also by providing community resources for aftercare and rehabilitation intended to facilitate discharges and to retain discharged patients in the community; while in Britain there has been increasing emphasis upon the preventive end of the spectrum, especially through encouraging construction of psychiatric facilities in general hospitals. But in balance, the approach in England remains primarily rehabilitative, while in the United States the stress upon primary prevention continues to dominate planning and programming.

The difference in program emphasis is reflected also in the other members of the mental health team. The occupational therapist in Britain has become increasingly concerned with industrial rehabilitation techniques rather than the more conventional occupational therapy activities, but otherwise she is probably the member of the team closest to her American counterpart. The clinical psychologist, so familiar and vital a participant in the United States, has been, until quite recently, a rarity in Britain. Such clinical psychologists as were available tended to work in mental institutions where their function was chiefly limited to diagnostic testing. Most British psychologists involved in community mental health activities have been "educational psychologists," based chiefly in child guidance clinics, whose work has been with children with behavioral disturbances. Their duties have included therapy as well as assessment. The psychiatric nurse in Britain has usually received training in a mental hospital only and has not had a general nursing background. There are many male mental nurses, while there are very few male general nurses. Their orientation has often remained rather traditional and concerned with maintenance of social skills, assessment of pathology, and administration of medications. The American psychiatric nurse is often more comfortable in a general hospital setting than is her British counterpart. In some quarters in England it has become quite fashionable for the psychiatric nurse to work in the community, making domiciliary visits. This usually involves follow-up of discharged former inpatients for the purpose of functional assessment, or to administer long-acting phenothiazines. Nurses also make home calls to check up on patients who have failed to come in for scheduled day-hospital sessions. Such practices have to a degree begun to be emulated in the United States but on a much smaller scale.

Social work in the United States has for many years been a professional calling, requiring graduate education at a Master's level, whereas in Britain, until fairly recently, the background of those calling themselves social workers has been extremely varied. Social workers in psychiatric institutions have functioned largely as history-takers; there usually were no more than one or two for a large hospital, so that many hospital-based psychiatrists have not been truly familiar with ways of fully utilizing social service skills in behalf of their patients. Social workers in community settings have been traditionally concerned with personal social services. Hence they are likely to be responsible for "case work" with many individual problems that in the United States would be handled psychotherapeutically by a psychiatrist. The need to establish normative educational standards and professional identity in social work led to a move in Britain to develop a separate Department of Social Services, which has removed the social worker from membership in clinical teams led by physicians.

Not only do the roles of treatment team members familiar to Americans differ, but in addition, Britain has categories of care-givers unfamiliar to the United States, such as the Mental Welfare Officer and the Disablement Resettlement Officer. The very existence of these categories tends to promote differences in patterns of delivery of mental health services.

The Mental Welfare Officer (MWO) is historically a statutory position within the local health authority. The MWO is responsible, among other things, for facilitating admission of patients to mental hospitals and often serves as liaison between the general practitioner and the psychiatrist. Traditionally the MWO concerned himself with community facilities and programs primarily for the mentally retarded, but the tendency has grown for involvement as well in community aftercare efforts in behalf of the mentally ill. While there were no special training requirements, many MWOs were former mental nurses. Increasingly, it became the practice in many local authorities to assign the functions of the MWOs to psychiatric social workers.

Following implementation of the Seebohm Report in 1971 (101), all former MWOs, whether or not they had been social workers, were absorbed into the new unified Social Service Department. Now the MWOs are expected to perform as "generic social workers" side by side with the others. The functions of the MWO are assigned to members of the Social Service Department usually without regard for whether or not the worker has had training in psychiatry or mental health. (See chapters 2 and 4.)

The Disablement Resettlement Officer (DRO) is an employee of what was formerly the Ministry of Labour but what is now called the Department of Employment and Productivity. His place on the mental health team comes by virtue of his important role in placing discharged mental patients into industrial jobs in the community. By visiting the industrial therapy workshops of the mental hospitals he familiarizes himself with the patients' work potentials prior to discharge, and he maintains active follow-up contacts after the patient begins working until he is satisfied that the job placement has been successful. His function is directly tied to the rehabilitation emphasis which characterizes British community psychiatry.

Efforts at assessment and evaluation of the effectiveness of British mental health services could have bearing on program development in the United States, provided fundamental differences between the two systems are clear. In Britain, for example, the major criterion of effectiveness has been social competence, as determined by community adjustment, ability to hold a job, capacity for independent responsibility, etc. Patients may be free of overt symptoms yet be considered a therapeutic failure because of an inability to work or live independently; while others may have persistent psychotic manifestations, yet be considered successfully treated, because they are able to live with their families and hold a job.

In the United States, on the other hand, there has been less emphasis on functioning capacity and a greater emphasis upon the existence of psychotic symptomatology. This difference in emphasis is also reflected in the different diagnostic approaches of psychiatrists in the two countries.

Several studies have attempted to assess the effectiveness, according to their criteria, of British programs heralded as "outstanding." So-called outstanding programs do not seem to be significantly different in their effectiveness from other programs of good quality. The programs receiving greatest attention are generally those whose leaders are skilled promoters. While their enthusiasm does tend to rub off on others, resulting in high morale and a feeling on the part of the mental health staff that they are performing worthwhile functions, it is not necessarily reflected in more successful treatment results. Furthermore, programs reflect the individuals responsible for creating them rather than the staff or the setting in which they are carried out, and tend to change when the person responsible for them moves to another position.

Adequacy of treatment for both the older and younger age

groups remains an unsolved problem. Accumulation of elderly patients in mental hospitals has threatened to undermine efforts to reduce the number of occupied inpatient beds, and has stimulated the development of special geriatric hospitals containing so-called "psycho-geriatric units" for the mentally-ill aged patient. Other approaches have included elaborate programs to maintain old people in the community as long as possible, with the aid of day centers, day hospitals, "Holiday care," etc. The latter is a program whereby the hospital temporarily admits the patient, who is otherwise cared for at home by his family, for brief periods to give family members some respite from the burdens of looking after him. The hospital accepts the patient on condition that the relatives will resume their responsibility within a specified time, or after a domestic crisis has passed. Patients will, of course, also be readmitted to the hospital if their condition deteriorates to a point where they are no longer manageable at home.

Programs for children are fragmented. Child guidance clinics and special schools for emotionally disturbed children are operated by the Local Authority Education Department, usually unrelated to any of the other community mental health efforts. Some children with behavior disorders are treated in psychiatric settings, organized along "family" lines. There are a few special units for autistic children in hospitals or day hospitals, but there is no coordinated program for their care, nor is their treatment in any way related to the programs for other emotionally disturbed children (60). Programs for the mentally retarded are also distinct, though they tend to be much better coordinated than those for mentally ill children. Hardly any resources for adolescents are to be found anywhere, although a few experimental pilot units have been opened or are about to open.

In Britain, community mental health services have for the most part evolved over the years in a rather haphazard fashion, ever since mental hospital services were first incorporated into the National Health Service in 1946.

Beginning in 1962, with the Hospital Plan for England and Wales (50), the Ministry of Health attempted to bring some order to the situation (described in greater detail in Chapter 3). Yet other events, such as the reorganization of the London boroughs (1964) and the continuing failure of local authorities to provide adequate facilities for community care for the mentally ill, as well as the unsolved problem of mentally ill chidren and senior citizens, prevented a comprehensive organization of community mental health services. Implementation of the Seebohm Report (101), which created the new Social Service Department outside the medical orbit, further weakened plans to provide comprehensive community mental health services. In the offing, however, is the implementation of several reports which should have a more stabilizing effect, despite the fact that each brings its own problems. These are the Todd Report (57) on medical education, the Redcliffe-Maud Report (58) on the reorganization of local governments and redesign of their boundaries, and the White Paper (59) on the reorganization of the National Health Service.

The Todd Report is a proposal to reorganize the present medical school curriculum by, among other things, placing less emphasis on the basic sciences, such as anatomy and physiology, and giving greater emphasis to the social and behavioral sciences. This should have the effect of improving the physician's appreciation of problems related to mental health. This is discussed further in Chapter 4.

The Redcliffe-Maud Report will alter the pattern of local government in England by changing the geographic boundaries of the present counties and boroughs. Thus, new local authorities will be created. The Ministry of Health's White Paper seeks to eliminate the tripartite structure of the National Health Service and to establish new area health authorities, which will correspond in number and area to the new local authorities. The reorganization of the National Health Service and the implications of these legislative changes are discussed in Chapters 2 and 3.

Finally, community mental health in Britain has approached a major crossroad. All of these changes have significant implications for the future directions of community mental health programs. What their ultimate influence will be remains for the future to determine, but they are bound to change the pattern and nature of existing programs. An attempt to assess some of these implications will be found in the Afterword.

2

The National Health Service

In order to understand the British system of mental health care, we should know something of the nature and organization of the National Health Service. The National Health Service in England and Wales was established by the National Health Service Act of 1946 and came into force on July 5, 1948 (35, 37). Corresponding legislation in Scotland and Northern Ireland established similar programs in these countries.

Under the health service scheme, a comprehensive range of health and welfare services is made available free of charge to all residents in Britain (34). Even visitors from abroad may receive free treatment if they fall ill during a visit. Almost everyone in Britain in every social class utilizes the health service.

Participation in the health service by the medical and allied professions is on a voluntary basis; however, the great majority of specialists and almost all of the general practitioners participate. The general consensus of attitude among the medical profession toward the health service is quite positive, in contrast to what many of us in the United States may have been led to believe. To be sure, there are many criticisms of various facets of its operation, and there are currently efforts to reorganize the health service. However, the aim is to improve, not to abolish it.

The Minister of Health is responsible for the administration of the National Health Service. As presently organized, the Ministry of Health is

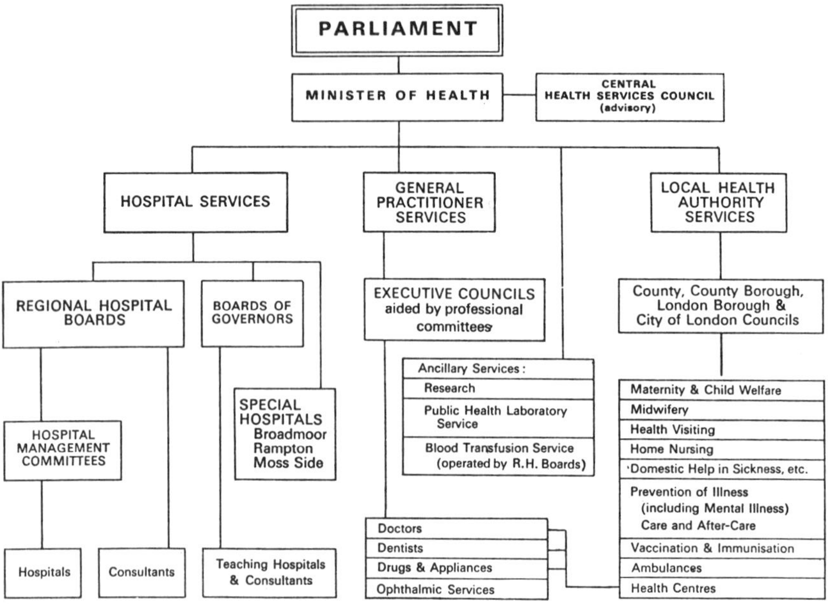

Organization of the National Health Service in England and Wales

The services in Scotland and Northern Ireland are somewhat differently organized. In Scotland the responsible Minister is the Secretary of State for Scotland, and in Northern Ireland the Minister of Health and Social Services.

"tripartite." That is, there are three main branches, each of which operates fairly independently of the others. These are the General Practitioner Services, the Local Authority Health Services, and the Hospital and Consultant, or Specialist, Services.

GENERAL PRACTITIONER SERVICES

The General Practitioner Services include dental, pharmaceutical, and ophthalmic services as well as the family doctor service. But the basic element of the health service is the family doctor (34). There are 21,500 general practitioners in England and Wales in the health service responsible to the Ministry of Health through 134 executive councils.

Patients may choose whichever general practitioner they wish, subject to the acceptance of the patient by the doctor, who is paid according to the number of patients on his list. The average list contains about 2,500 patients. The maximum allowable is 3,500.

LOCAL AUTHORITY HEALTH SERVICES

The second pillar of the National Health Service tripartite is the Local Authority Health Service. The term "local authority" applies to the various units of the local government in England and Wales. There are presently 174 Local Health Authorities (34).*

Local Authority Health Services include care of mothers and young children, family planning, domiciliary midwife services, health visiting, home nursing, vaccination and immunization, prevention of illness, care and aftercare, home helps, ambulance service, and establishment of health centers. In addition, under the National Assistance Act of 1948, local authorities are responsible for providing a number of welfare and social services including residential accommodations, temporary accommodations for people in urgent need, services for the elderly in their own homes, including "meals on wheels," and services for the handicapped, including those suffering from mental disorders.

Local Health Authorities have statutory responsibility to make

*The Redcliffe-Maud Report (58), which will go into effect in 1974, recommends that England be divided into 61 new local government areas, instead of the existing 174. In 58 of these areas, a single authority is to be responsible for all services for a population ranging from 250,000 to 1,000,000. In the three large metropolitan areas around Birmingham, Liverpool, and Manchester, responsibility for such services will be divided between a metropolitan authority whose key function is planning transportation and major development, and a number of metropolitan district authorities which are concerned with education, the personal social services, health, and housing.

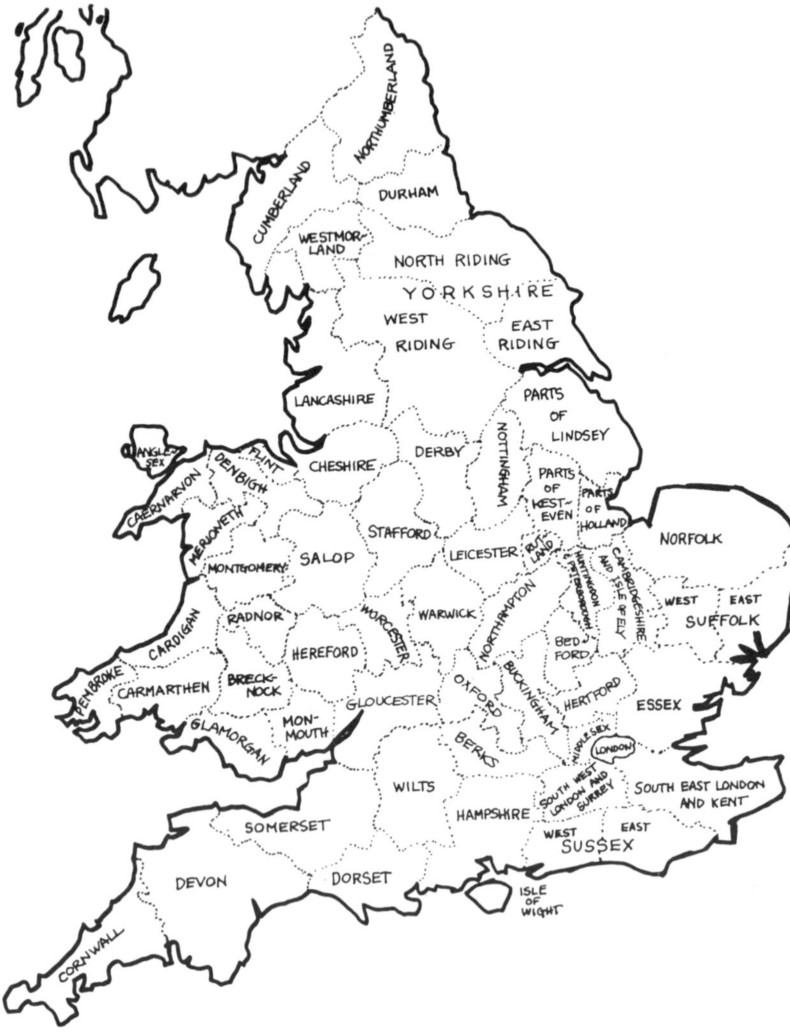

Local Health Authorities and Executive Councils

As of 1973, 174 local health authorities, 58 county councils, 82 county boroughs, the 32 London boroughs, the city of London, and the Isles of Scilly are responsible for all local health authority services in England and Wales; 134 executive councils are responsible for the family practitioner service.

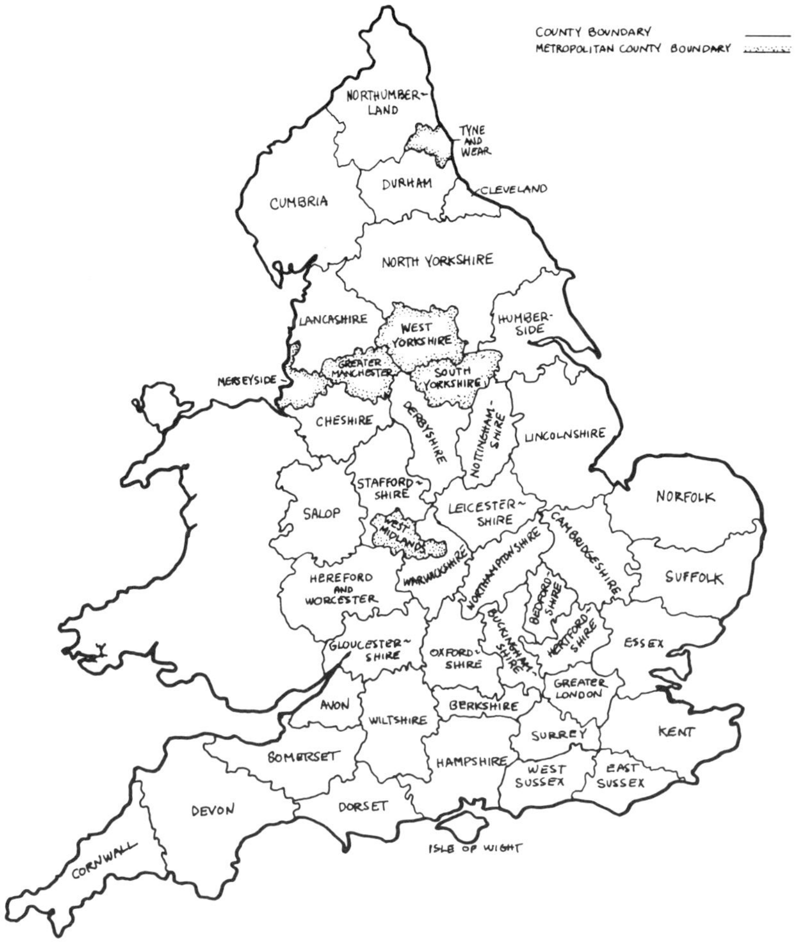

Reorganization of local authorities pursuant to the Redcliffe-Maud Report (effective April 1974.)

arrangements for the prevention of mental illness, the care of people suffering from any form of mental disorder, and their aftercare. These arrangements include provisions of suitable residential accommodations such as hostels for those who do not need to enter the hospital or for those unable to be discharged until they have somewhere to go where they can receive continuing help. They also are expected to smooth the return to full everyday responsibilities after a period of hospital treatment.

The Chief Medical Officer of the local authority, called the Medical Officer of Health (MOH), is a physician, generally with training in public health. He is chief administrative officer of the Local Authority Health Department and has the statutory duty to ascertain, report, and advise upon all conditions that affect the health of the community. The major concern of the MOH has been the control of communicable diseases by improvement of environmental health, especially in such areas as water supply, refuse and sewage disposal, and housing. In recent years, many of these duties have been taken up by specially trained experts such as sanitary engineers, water engineers, and experts in planning and housing. As a consequence, the areas of responsibility of the MOH have become progressively narrowed.

For many of the MOHs, the local authority responsibilities in the area of community mental health were a major area of interest and concern. In many communities the MOH put a great deal of his energies and his budget into the development of a strong mental health section within the Local Authority Health Department.

When the Seebohm Report (101) was implemented in 1971, however, the social work staff of the mental health section was transferred to the new Social Service Department further limiting the scope of responsibility and the size of the budget of the MOH. As a consequence many of the MOHs have not taken kindly to the new department. In many cases there is a significant power struggle between the MOH and the new Social Service director. In a few instances, such as in Croydon and Camden, the MOH has managed to remain on good terms with the director, and in Newham, the MOH was appointed as the director of the Social Service Department.

The future of the MOH is an uncertain one. Now called the Community Physician, he continues to have important responsibilities in the areas of communicable disease control, vaccination and immunization, and enforcement responsibilities relating to working conditions affecting health, epidemiology, and health education (40). For all local authorities except Birmingham, the MOH has also served as Chief Medical Officer of the Education Department. However, it is not clear where responsibility for school health will be placed following the reorganization of the health services, nor what duties will remain in the hands of the Community Physician.

In addition to providing schooling for normal children, the Education Department maintains special schools for handicapped children, including those who are mentally disturbed, and also operates child guidance clinics. The MOH continues to be responsible for providing medical services to the special schools and guidance clinics and frequently employs a child psychiatrist as consultant. Most of the therapeutic work in these schools or clinics, however, is done by educational psychologists.

Under the present rather topsy-turvy system, guidance clinics and special schools for mentally disturbed children are the responsibility of the Local Authority Education Department, while the Local Health Authority has been responsible for the mentally retarded children and adults. The Local Health Authority was required to provide special schools, hostels, and other facilities for the care of both subnormal and severely subnormal people of all ages, as well as providing services for mentally ill adults. These functions were generally administered through the mental health section of the health department but are now the responsibility of the Social Service Department. Following the reorganization of the health service in 1974, children's psychiatric clinics will be increasingly based at district general hospitals under medical auspices, while responsibility for the care of mentally subnormal children and adults will be moved to the Education Department.

A traditional statutory post in the mental health section has been that of the Mental Welfare Officer (MWO). This is a position descended from the old "overseer of the poor" under Elizabethan poor laws. In recent years the MWO has had responsibility for seeing that the mentally retarded were properly cared for, responsibility for expediting admission of the mentally ill to mental hospitals, and certain responsibilities for aftercare as well. There were no special training requirements for the job, although the MWO was often trained as a mental nurse. When the Chidren's Department, Welfare Department, and mental health section of the Health Department were unified to form the Local Authority Social Service Department, all of the MWOs, whether or not they had been social workers, were included in the new Department. The MWOs are now considered "generic social workers," and the functions of the MWO are now assigned to all members of the Social Service Department, regardless of whether they have had a background in psychiatry or mental health. (See "Social Work," Chapter 4.)

HOSPITAL AND CONSULTANT SERVICES

Hospital and Consultant services form the third major pillar of the National Health Service. There are today over 2,500 hospitals in England and Wales, including 26 London and 12 provincial teaching hospi-

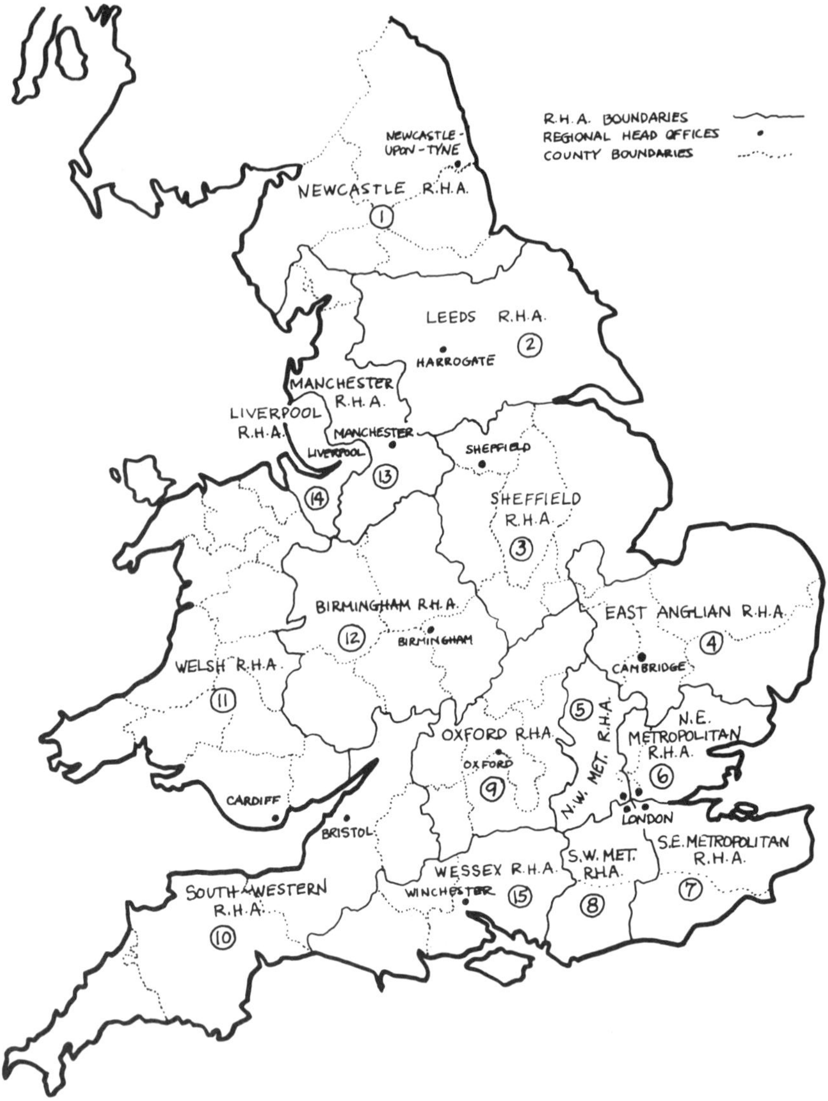

Regional Hospital Areas in England and Wales

England and Wales are divided into 14 regional hospital areas, as of 1973.

tals. They comprise over 434,000 beds. Almost one-half of the beds (47%) are psychiatric, distributed among 150 mental hospitals (83). Relatively few hospitals remain outside of the health service, and these are generally run by religious orders.

England is currently divided into 14 hospital regions, each with a regional hospital board responsible to the Ministry of Health for planning and coordinating the Hospital and Consultant (Specialist) services in the non-teaching hospitals. The actual administration of the individual hospitals or groups of hospitals is carried out by 330 hospital management committees, responsible to their respective 14 regional hospital boards (34). These committees have responsibility for the day-to-day operation of the hospitals and for the appointments of all staff except senior medical and dental staff.

While the medical community has not shown a readiness to do away with the socialized-medicine system, there certainly have been frequent, vigorous criticisms of various aspects of the program as it has been organized. The lack of uniform development of community facilities by the local authorities, the division of responsibility for mental health programs between the local authorities and the mental hospitals, and the lack of continuity of care are some of the difficulties encountered by psychiatrists. These, as well as similar problems in other areas finally made it clear that there was a need to reorganize the structure of the National Health Service (see the National Health Service after Reorganization).

The Hospital Services provide for all forms of care and treatment in specialized and general hospitals. Besides the mental hospitals, there are a number of hospitals especially for children, in addition to some children's wards in general hospitals.

The teaching hospitals, which provide the undergraduate and postgraduate medical education and therefore are affiliated with medical schools, are not under regional hospital boards but have their own boards of governors directly responsible to the Ministry of Health. However, there is at least one teaching hospital in each hospital region.

The vast majority of specialists, called "consultants" in Britain, participate in the health service and maintain appointments at particular hospitals. Neither the specialist nor the general practitioner is prevented from accepting private patients, but they must be on a part-time arrangement to do so. The salary scale in 1970 was between $8,300 and $12,600 per year for a full-time hospital consultant. There are, however, certain additional forms of remuneration that may more than double that income.

The scales of remuneration of consultants and other doctors and dentists are based on recommendations made by the Review Body which was set up in March 1962 to advise the Prime Minister on the remuneration of doctors and dentists in the National Health Service (36). The

Review Body awards additional remuneration to consultants in the form of distinction awards and extra duty payments. Distinction awards are given to those who have made a special contribution to medicine or for outstanding professional work, and extra duty payments are awarded to consultants for additional work outside of the hospital, such as domiciliary visits. This is discussed further in Chapter 4.

The Review Body's Report recommended a general increase of 30% in the remuneration of hospital doctors and dentists for two years beginning April 1, 1970 (36, 38, 55). When the report was published on June 4, 1970, the government announced acceptance of this recommendation for the training grades but referred half the recommended increase for the career grades to the National Board for Prices and Incomes (NBPI) for further advice. This decision was followed by the resignation of the members of the Review Body. It also led the British Medical Association to advise doctors not to sign national insurance medical certificates, and, together with the British Dental Association, to call for a withdrawal of cooperation by doctors and dentists in National Health Service Administration. The government fell soon afterward, and a new election was held. After the general election these sanctions were lifted in return for an assurance from the new government that the reference of the increase to the NBPI would be withdrawn and a new independent Review Body set up. On August 7, the government announced its decision to settle the pay of the career grades for one year only and for this period to limit the increase to 5% over the 1969 levels, the increase above the 15% already awarded by the previous government (38).

There are about 2,800 psychiatrists in the Hospital Service. Slightly more than 1,000 of them are consultants or fully qualified specialists. The others have a lesser status, many of them in training positions equivalent to residency. Only the fully accredited specialists may see private patients.

Most consultant psychiatrists work in the mental hospitals. A number of them hold joint appointments; that is, in addition to their mental hospital post, they may hold appointments with a general hospital psychiatry department, with a teaching hospital, with a local authority, or with some combination of these. There are few full-time teaching positions for psychiatrists since psychiatry is not emphasized in the medical schools.

Every person is enrolled with a general practitioner who is responsible for that individual's general health. Illnesses which the general practitioner can care for personally, he treats himself. If the patient requires hospitalization or specialized services, the general practitioner refers the patient to a consultant at an appropriate hospital.

If the patient suffers from a mental illness, the general practitioner will tend to call in the mental welfare officer (formerly a member of the staff of the Local Health Authority but now on the staff of the Social Service Department), who is available 24 hours a day, 7 days per week. After the MWO has ascertained the general nature of the problem, he or she will arrange either for the patient to be evaluated at an outpatient clinic, or for the psychiatric consultant to visit the patient at his home. If admission to the hospital is decided upon, the patient will usually be under the care of the consultant who did the evaluation.

The psychiatrist may decide against admission, in which event he may return the patient to the care of his general practitioner with advice for further treatment. He may arrange for the patient to be seen at an outpatient clinic for ambulatory electroconvulsive therapy (ECT),* or other treatment; or he may refer the patient to whatever local-authority services may be available, such as day centers, sheltered workshops, or therapeutic social clubs.

After treatment in a mental hospital, a patient may be referred to a day hospital, industrial rehabilitation unit, or other post-hospital rehabilitation facility operated by the hospital itself; or he may be referred for aftercare to the local authority services; or he may be returned to the care of his general practitioner.

THE NATIONAL HEALTH SERVICE AFTER REORGANIZATION

The need for modifying the organization of the National Health Service has long been recognized. Toward this end the government issued a Green Paper in 1968 proposing certain changes. The reaction of the medical community to this document was almost entirely negative, however, and a second Green Paper (40) was issued in 1970.

The response to this document was somewhat more positive, and finally a White Paper (59) was issued in 1972, which outlined a program of reorganization intended to form a more unified and integrated service. Basically, the new plan will eliminate the tripartite structure of the National Health Service. A key feature of the reorganization plan is its integration with the planned reorganization of local governments (58) scheduled to take place in April 1974. The health service reorganization has been timed to coincide with this.

The key term of the reorganized National Health Service is "administrative unification." The services that will be brought together under the unified National Health Service administration include: the hospital and specialist services now administered by the regional hospital boards, hospital management committees, and boards of governors; the

*This term is used synonomously with the term electroshock therapy (EST) in the text.

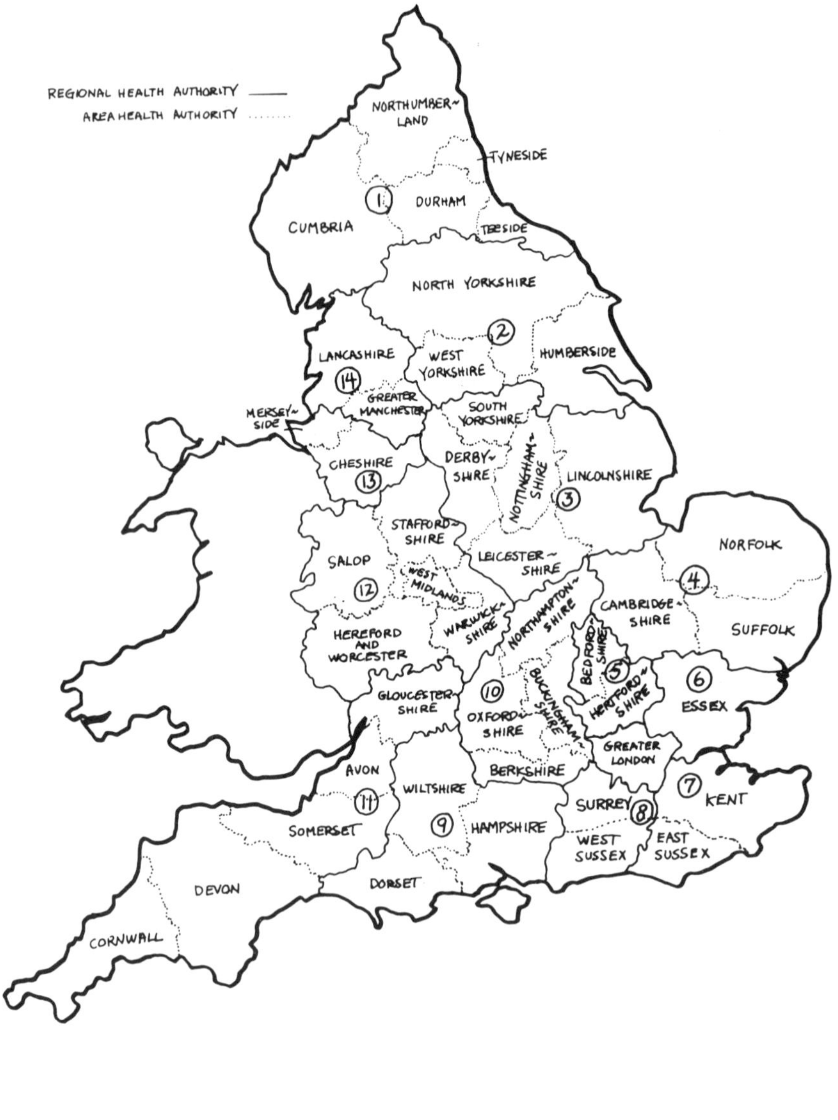

Regional health authorities and area health authorities following the reorganization of the National Health Service to be implemented in 1974.

family practitioner services now administered by the executive councils; the personal health services now administered by the local authorities; and the school health services. The personal health services are ambulance services; epidemiology work; family planning; health centers; health visiting; home nursing and midwifery; maternity and child health care; medical, nursing, and supplementary arrangements for the prevention of illness; care and aftercare (including mental illness); and vaccination and immunization. The registration of nursing homes will also become the responsibility of the National Health Service.

At present the Local Education Authorities are responsible for school, medical, and dental services. This responsibility will be transferred to the National Health Service, which will make available to Local Education Authorities medical, dental, nursing, and allied resources which the education authorities may need to carry out their responsibility of education of handicapped and disabled children. Similarly, "child guidance" functions currently carried out by the Local Education Authorities will be transferred to children's psychiatric clinics to be based at district general hospitals.

The personal social services will continue to be the responsibility of the Local Authority Social Service Department. Hospital social workers will be transferred to the Local Authority Social Services Department on April 1, 1974. Thus, a dichotomization of two important elements of community mental health remains despite the "unification" watchword of the White Paper. (The social workers are not a part of the National Health Service but instead, are responsible to the local authority or local government.) Environmental health will also continue to be a function of local government. This includes prevention of communicable diseases; food safety; port health; animal diseases, insofar as they affect human health; job health aspects of environmental services; and enforcement of proper environmental conditions at places of work.

Administration of the National Health Service will be delegated to local bodies. These will be at two levels, regional and area, in addition to the central department. At each level will be a unified administrative structure covering all responsibilities of the National Health Service. Each Area Health Authority (AHA) will serve the same population within the same boundaries as its matching local authority established pursuant to the Redcliffe-Maud recommendations (58). Hopefully this will make it easier for collaboration to occur when there are areas of overlap between responsibilities of the local authorities and responsibilities of the National Health Service. A case in point would be community mental health programs.

The central department of the National Health Service will set national health policies. The Regional Health Authorities (RHAs) will have regional planning responsibilities including the setting of priorities and resolving competing claims between areas. The area health authorities will make plans for the communities within the areas–the "districts,"–and this is expected to wield a strong influence on the establishment of local, regional, and national priorities. It is expected that the AHA will plan and develop its service in consultation with its matching local authority and with the RHA. The Area Health Authority will also be an operator of services; it will employ the staff working at area headquarters and in the districts. Initially, however, consultants and senior registrars (except those in teaching hospitals) will continue to be appointed at the regional level. The AHA will also be responsible for the supporting services needed to back up delivery of comprehensive health care.

Day-to-day operation of services will be "district" based. Each district will contain a district general hospital or several hospitals and will cover a population of 200,000 to 500,000 people. The district boundaries will not necessarily correspond to local government districts. Many AHAs will encompass only one or two districts; a few will have as many as five. The districts will not form a separate tier of authority but will simply provide a pattern of organization for delivery of health care to the population. The 32 London boroughs and the city of London will be grouped to form a smaller number of health areas. Outside of London there will be identities between health areas and local authority areas; consequently, there will be 72 AHAs outside of London.

The general medical and dental practitioners, ophthalmologists, opticians, and pharmacists will continue to serve as independent contractors, as they do now. However, they will no longer be responsible to the executive councils. Instead, each Area Health Authority will set up a Family Practitioner Committee (FPC) which will enter into contracts with the individual practitioners. Remuneration patterns will be set nationally. On these matters the Family Practitioner Committee will deal directly with the central health department; otherwise the committee will be responsible to the AHA.

The Area Health Authorities in turn will be responsible to the Regional Health Authorities. Each region will have a university medical school within its boundaries. It is expected that there will be 14 health regions corresponding to the 14 hospital regions currently used. Each region will contain a number of complete health areas, and no health area will be broken up between more than one region.

Some of the Area Health Authorities will contain teaching hospitals (medical schools). They will be known as "teaching areas" [AHA(T)s]. The teaching areas will be administered as part of the regions in which they are located, but a close relationship will probably be maintained by the AHA(T) and the teaching hospital administration.

Those currently known as medical officers of health (MOHs) will be redesignated as "specialists in community medicine" and will function through the area, region, and central department hierarchical structure. While their ultimate function is still unclear, an attempt at some definition of their duties has been made in the Report of the Working Party on Medical Administrators (43).

Plans are being made to facilitate the implementation of the reorganization on April 1, 1974. Undoubtedly many transitional problems will arise, and several administrative schemes have been established to cope with these problems.

3

The roots of the community mental health program

THE DEVELOPMENT OF HEALTH SERVICES IN BRITAIN

Contrary to popular misconception in the United States, the present health care delivery system of Britain (i.e., the so-called "socialized medicine") did not come about as a consequence of revolutionary innovation, but developed rather as the product of a gradual evolution, having its roots as far back as the Middle Ages.

In medieval times various town councils had responsibility for issuing sanitary regulations for the protection of the public health. Care of the sick, including the indigent sick, was usually the responsibility of the monasteries, which established the hospitals which were the forerunners of the voluntary hospitals of today (35).

During the reign of Henry VIII, when the national religion of Britain was changed from Catholic to Protestant, the monasteries were abolished, and most of the hospitals founded by the monastic orders died out. To care for the sick poor left without health resources by the dissolution of the monasteries, a system of "poor-law hospitals" was established during the reign of Queen Elizabeth I. Such poor-law hospitals and workhouses spread throughout the country during the next three-and-a-half centuries, caring for the indigent. These hospitals were the ancestors of the municipal hospitals of today.

Conditions of hospital wards for the destitute sick were often deplorable, and during the 18th and 19th centuries, in a climate of social reform, there was a renewed emphasis on the founding of voluntary hospitals. Most of the big London hospitals existing today were founded and endowed by local citizens during this time as charitable institutions for the sick and poor.

During the 19th century the industrial revolution caused a rapid growth of towns, thus creating urgent sanitary problems. The Public Health Act of 1848 attempted to set a common minimum standard of sanitation and provided for supervision of local public health standards by a central board. This act required local authorities to appoint medical officers of health and public health inspectors. This law has been updated and consolidated by subsequent legislation, but not markedly changed to the present day, so that local authorities continue to have extensive powers for making and administering local laws relating to public health.

During the latter 19th and early 20th centuries some effort was made to improve poor-law institutions. The need for such improvement became all the more important following the inauguration of the National Health Insurance scheme in 1912. However, these efforts did not succeed too well, so that by 1930, administrative responsibility for poor-law institutions and workhouses was transferred from the Poor Law Board of Guardians to the local authorities, specifically to the county and borough councils. These councils were given power to take over workhouse wards and run them as ordinary general hospitals, and many councils did so. By 1939 London, Manchester, Birmingham, Middlesex, and other councils had taken over workhouse infirmaries and had upgraded them so that many of these hospitals rivaled voluntary hospitals in the same area.

Thus, most communities had two types of hospitals: one, a voluntary hospital at which the medical staff was "voluntary" or unpaid, and the other, a municipal or poor-law hospital, the staff of which was salaried. Around 60% of the nation's beds were in the municipal hospitals.

When the National Health Service came into being in 1948, almost all hospitals, voluntary as well as municipal, were taken into this system. Still, the provision of hospital services over the country was uneven in both quality and quantity. Many hospitals were small with limited facilities, and most were housed in old, inconvenient buildings. Efforts to improve the situation were hampered by limitations of capital funds, and until 1955 most of these efforts were directed towards improving existing institutions. In 1956, however, the nation embarked on an expanded hospital-building program, and in 1962 the government published long range plans for modernization of hospital services, including an accelerated program of hospital construction. This plan was updated in 1966 to cover the decade 1966–76 (52).

THE DEVELOPMENT OF THE MENTAL HEALTH SERVICES

The British community mental health program as it exists today likewise evolved gradually over a number of years. Thus, there was no overall plan but rather an accumulation of bits and pieces with periodic attempts to formalize and coordinate them by acts of Parliament.

The first legislation dealing specifically with mental illness was the Lunacy Act of 1890, which consolidated responsibility for establishing asylums for the insane. The main objective of this legislation was to protect the patient and society. The Victorian mental institutions constructed as a consequence of this Act tended, like their counterparts in the United States, to be large and built in the country away from centers of population. Patients were admitted to these hospitals by legal certification. The mental institutions were run by local authorities, and the patients had to pay charges according to their means or those of responsible relatives. The National Health Insurance scheme of 1912 did not cover mental illness.

A Mental Treatment Act was passed in 1930 which provided for voluntary admission of patients to mental hospitals and set up psychiatric outpatient clinics at general hospitals, at which psychiatrists from mental hospitals treated patients who were living at home (41).

The National Health Service Act of 1946, which was put into operation in 1948, finally brought mental hospitals into the comprehensive hospital scheme under the overall supervision of a Board of Control (46). The health scheme provided free treatment for psychiatric inpatients, although outpatients still had to pay a portion of the prescription charges for their medicines. The incorporation of the mental institutions within the orb of the other hospitals resulted in an effort to upgrade these overcrowded, run-down institutions and to increase the number of available beds. In addition, the establishment of the National Health Service gave to the Local Health Authorities statutory responsibility for providing mental health services in the areas of prevention and aftercare.

Following an extensive study of the problems of mental illness conducted by the Royal Commission on Mental Illness and Mental Deficiency (56), new mental health legislation was enacted. The Mental Health Act of 1959 repealed all prior mental health legislation and attempted to replace it with a coordinated set of regulations. There were two major emphases of this law. One was to stress informal (voluntary) admissions to hospitals and to simplify the procedure for hospitalization. The second was to shift emphasis in the treatment of psychiatric patients from the hospital to the community.

Although it emphasized informal admissions, the 1959 Mental Health Act did not neglect to provide for compulsory admission to mental hospitals. However, the law included safeguards against unnecessary detention through the establishment of special tribunals to which patients or their relatives might apply for review. The act also dissolved the Board of Control, vesting full authority over mental hospitals in the Ministry of Health. It removed previous requirements that mentally ill patients could be admitted to only specifically designated hospitals. This provided greater flexibility by permitting compulsory admission of patients to any hospital, including general hospitals. It also clarified the power of the local authorities by specifying the services to be provided by them, such as sheltered residential accommodations and training centers for mentally ill and mentally subnormal patients. It outlined procedures for guardianship and allowed services which had previously been provided for the physically handicapped under the National Assistance Act to be used in caring for the mentally ill in the community.

The effect of this legislation upon community care was actually to formalize a trend that had been developing in mental hospitals over a period of years. These institutions, large as they were, were becoming overcrowded as admission rates climbed steadily. Between 1949 and 1960 the annual rate of admissions to mental hospitals had more than doubled, rising from 55,000 to 114,000 (83).

One attempt to alleviate this situation was an effort to reduce the admission rate. A notable illustration of such an effort was the Worthing Experiment (10, 11, 12). Under this scheme, Dr. Joshua Carse, the medical superintendent of the Graylingwell Hospital in Chichester, visited in their own homes patients who had been referred for hospitalization. He would give treatment to the patients and advice to their families in the hope of enabling the patients to be cared for at home, thus avoiding admission to the hospital. This experimental approach was able in its final year to reduce admissions to Graylingwell by 59%, even prior to the general use of psychotropic drugs.

The significant reduction of mental hospital populations did not occur, however, until after the introduction of tranquilizers. In 1954, the year that phenothiazines were first used, the mental hospital population had reached a peak of 148,000 (83). By the following year, the number of occupied beds began to fall at the rate of 1,000 per year. The impact of tranquilizers encouraged hospitals to intensify their already vigorous efforts to mobilize chronic institutionalized patients and to discharge them to the community. Often ingenious programs of resocialization and rehabilitation were instituted. Greater emphasis was placed on outpatient treatment and day-hospital programs. By 1960, the number of patients in mental hospitals had been reduced to 135,000, a drop of 12,000 in five years (83).

The Hospital Plan for England and Wales (50), published in 1962, took note of this shift in emphasis. Based upon a study by Tooth and Brooke (106) of the trend towards reduction in the number of occupied mental hospital beds, the plan anticipated an increase in psychiatric treatment in regional general hospitals and in local authority programs and a reduction in the need for institutional beds from 147,000 in 1960 to 80,000 by 1975. This represented a decrease in the ratio of mental hospital beds to populations from 3.3 per 1,000 to 1.8 per 1,000 (106). While the plan anticipated a decrease in the number of long-stay mental patients, it expected that the number of short- and medium-stay patients would increase.

This anticipated bed reduction was not expected to be uniform (8). The plan called for the number of mental hospitals with 1,000 or more beds to be reduced from 69 to 26 but anticipated an increase in the number of psychiatric units in general hospitals from 82 to 168 by 1975. This represented an increase of 7,127 general hospital psychiatric beds. The overall reduction in psychiatric hospital beds expected, taking into account both mental and general hospitals, amounted to almost 40% (83).

Even though admission rates climbed steadily, the number of occupied beds continued to decline. Thus, by 1967, despite a record 185,000 admissions, there were fewer than 122,000 patients in the hospitals, and by 1968 this number was below 118,500 (53, 83). The key to the reduction in hospital population was the sharp increase in the discharge rate, which was climbing even faster than admission rates. Almost 6,000 more patients were discharged in 1968 than in 1967.

The rundown in occupied mental hospital beds meant, however, that programs of out-of-hospital care had to be developed. In some instances, hospitals maintained a continuing active interest in their former patients and played a prominent role in providing aftercare services such as outpatient clinics and day hospitals operated by mental hospital staffs; but for most patients, including thousands of discharged chronic institutionalized patients, provisions for employment, housing, and continuing care were expected to be developed by the local authorities (84). The burden of responsibility for the care of these patients was being shifted *de facto* from the hospitals to the communities.

While the hospital plan had indeed anticipated a sharp increase in construction of hostels for the mentally ill and provision of other services by the local authorities, the planners had no actual knowledge of what the local authorities really intended to do in this regard. It was not until 1963, a year after the publication of the Hospital Plan, that the Ministry of Health published a projected plan for the development of local authority community health and welfare services based on ten-year projections made by the various local authorities (51). This document anticipated an increase in the number of hostels for the mentally ill from 20 in 1963 to 240 by 1975 and an increase in the number of social workers on local authority staffs from 2,775 to 4,752. However, there were wide variations in the increments planned for by different local authorities. For example, Bedfordshire with a population in 1963 of over 400,000 had no mental health facilities at that time, and according to its plans as reported in the "Plans for the Health and Welfare Services for the Local Authorities" published in 1964, it intended to develop none through 1974. Somerset, with over half a million population, planned one occupational center providing 50 places and one hostel with 25 places, neither to be constructed until after 1970. Kent, with over 1 million people, planned only 3 hostels to provide 86 places. On the other hand, Essex, with a similar population, was planning 6 sheltered workshops to provide 176 places and 12 hostels to provide 294 places.

SOME PROBLEMS AND PARADOXES

Division of Responsibilities

While the Mental Health Act of 1959, intending to carry out the recommendations of the Royal Commission, defined the responsibilities of the local authorities for providing preventive and aftercare services for mentally ill patients, it paradoxically established, at the same time, a division of authority and responsibility for maintaining continuity of care.

One factor which in many instances interfered with the development of full cooperation and coordination between hospital and local authority was the differing extent of their respective catchment areas. The areas of responsibility for the particular units of local government were the geographical boundaries of the political subdivision. Hospital districts, on the other hand, might have no relationship whatsoever to these political lines, being based rather on the particular zone of responsibility historically assigned to the particular institution. Large mental hospitals might serve several small communities; whereas major population centers, such as London, required a number of mental hospitals, whose zones of responsibility might or might not coincide with the particular political subdivisions of the county boroughs.

The distribution of catchment areas was even further complicated following the reorganization of the London Boroughs in 1964. This reorganization altered boundaries, combined boroughs into new units, and created new boroughs where none had been before. It also complicated the projected plans of the local authorities in the London metropolitan area for development of community-based mental health facilities. Since the 1963 regional plans had been developed by political entities in existence prior to the reorganization, the boundaries and populations served were in many instances significantly altered.

Many areas of responsibility previously held by the London County Council were shifted to county boroughs following the reorganization. Local authority services are financed largely on income from "rates" or property taxes within the subdivision (subsidized by grants from the national treasury). Areas most impoverished, and therefore generally most in need of services, were also the areas with the lowest tax base and hence the least amount of available funds for providing needed facilities. Planning of "community care" was, of necessity, based upon anticipated income from particular localities, many of which were grossly changed in composition after the reorganization.

The reorganization also changed the make-up of the Borough Councils, the composition of which naturally determined the attitude of particular county boroughs towards provision for the mentally ill. For example, the Boroughs of East Ham and West Ham were combined by the reorganization into a single Borough of Newham. The two local authorities differed in make-up and attitude, and each had different emphases in the services provided. East Ham was more advanced in some areas, but West Ham was more progressive in the area of community mental health. The amalgamation was experienced as "a major convulsion," with each department fearing takeover by the other (73).

There was also unevenness in the legacy of facilities that had previously been developed by the London County Council, which had had the responsibility for providing these services prior to the reorganization. Some of the new boroughs found themselves with a number of existing and operating facilities of good quality and had a ready-made program to serve as a base for future development. Other boroughs, on the other hand, found that the areas they encompassed were devoid of such facilities.

Despite these handicaps, a number of heroic attempts have been made to find solutions to the problems. Many ingenious programs were developed by hospitals, by local authorities, or jointly between them, bridging statutory gaps by human enterprise. Some of the local authorities took the initiative in providing community facilities for aftercare and rehabilitation of patients discharged from mental hospitals, carried out with minimal assistance or communication from the hospital itself; on the other hand, services were developed which were primarily extensions into the community of those offered by the hospitals, with minimal support contributions from the local authorities. Fortunately there were, in addition, several efforts at cooperative action between hospitals and local authorities to provide services that were coordinated and integrated in varying degrees. Such services were usually based upon the development of schemes for making joint appointments of psychiatric consultants to the local authorities as well as to the mental hospital. Similar joint appointments were also extended to social workers in a number of instances.

The development of psychiatric units in general hospitals likewise provided opportunity for joint participation between local authorities and psychiatric facilities. However, each joint arrangement was unique and reflected the personality and conception of the individuals in charge of developing such programs. Not only did they fail to serve as general models for a national community mental health program; they tended to break down when the originator of the arrangement retired or accepted appointment elsewhere.

Nevertheless, there have been a number of attempts by the government to initiate programs and to formulate policies on a more rational basis than in the past. By November 1969, a Hospital Advisory Service was instituted, its first task being to inquire into the "long-stay" mental hospitals (39). Reports of this body indicated the need for more comprehensive planning, and in April 1971, the government asked the Regional Hospital Boards to provide additional details of hospital services provided for the mentally ill. The outcome was a government plan, formulated in January 1972, to establish minimum standards for "certain categories of staff and amenities for existing mental hospitals" (88). This at least reflected an increased interest by the Health Ministry in improving standards and restructuring services of mental hospitals.

Another effort to bring direction to the development of mental health services was the promulgation by the Health Ministry of a memorandum on Hospital Services for the Mentally Ill (42), which recommended that psychiatric units be provided in every district general hospital. These services were intended to include inpatient, day-hospital, and outpatient facilities for adults residing in the district. The memorandum also included guidelines for a "Standard Psychiatric Department" based on a common design plan but adapted to the particular conditions prevailing at individual hospitals. The overall program design called for multidisciplinary teams, including doctors, nurses, social workers, psychologists, and "where possible," the patient's general practitioner. Such teams were to be developed not only at general hospital departments of psychiatry, but at mental hospitals as well.

Another suggested innovation was the reorganization of the mental hospitals into "divisions," each to correspond to a particular catchment area it is to serve. The ultimate objective was to close down the mental hospitals as soon as possible. It was expected that as soon as psychiatric departments were available in the district general hospital, admissions to the mental hospital for that district would cease, although it was anticipated that clinical teams would be required to remain active at the mental hospital to care for chronically ill patients already there. It was hoped, however, that even these patients might ultimately be sent out for community care when adequate hostels, day centers, and community occupational facilities were available (42).

The very young and the very old patient remain a problem. The aged were to be hospitalized in special geriatric departments in general hospitals (88). Such hospitalization was to be for assessment rather than care. Alternatively, such assessment might be carried out at home, or on an outpatient, or day-patient basis.

Fragmentation of Child Psychiatric Services

The National Health Service Act of 1946 assigned to the Health Service responsibility for treating psychiatric disorders in children as well as adults (46). A Health Ministry memorandum in 1947 (49), and a complementary circular issued by the Ministry of Education in 1948 (47) seemed to establish quite clearly that clinical services relating to "children suffering from mental illness and maladjustment" were the responsibility of the Regional Hospital Boards, while the local authority was expected to provide services related to educational problems. Had these initial clear delineations of responsibilities been followed, it is likely that the subsequent fragmentation of children's psychiatric services would not have occurred.

In fact, however, these pronouncements were unrealizable. Child psychiatry was by no means a well-established discipline, and clinical psychiatric services for children were only slowly being developed. Another problem was semantic. Many child psychiatric problems were considered "maladjustments" rather than clinical entities, and it was erroneously believed that childhood psychosis was the main concern of the child psychiatrist; even the Royal Medico-Psychological Association took this view, with the 1957 publication: Memorandum on the Committee on Maladjusted Children, which stated, "To regard 'maladjustment' in a child as a clinical entity is inaccurate—the obsessional child . . . and the child liable to psychotic outburst do not represent the same entities" (68). The bulk of services for "maladjusted" children had been provided previously by "child guidance clinics" operated largely by the local authorities. Thus in 1950 a Committee on Maladjusted Children was set up by the Ministry of Education, "To inquire into . . . problems relating to maladjusted children, with reference to their treatment within the educational system" (68). The Committee Report (48), issued in 1955, advocated establishment of "joint clinics," that is, under joint local authority and health service auspices. Non-psychiatric staff and physical facilities were to be provided by the Local Authority Education Department, the School Health Service, and the Public Health Service. The psychiatrist was to be furnished by the Hospital Service.

In consequence, services developed haphazardly and sometimes at cross purposes. Roles were unclear: the educational psychologist sometimes took on medical functions, and even the clinical "team" headed by the child psychiatrist failed to make clear who was to be responsible for what (68).

During the interim between the committee's appointment and its report, however, child psychiatry programs under medical auspices had been developing, and the report was viewed as a regressive step by the British Pediatric Association, the British Medical Association, and the Royal Medico-Psychological Association (68). The BMA appointed a special subcommittee on child psychiatric services which recommended that such services be hospital based, a view endorsed by a 1962 Review of Medical Services in Great Britain (68).

It was gradually becoming more feasible to implement such recommendations. Whereas there had only been 64 hospital-based child psychiatric clinics in the country in 1956, only five years later there were 102, which included 72 at general hospitals, 17 at childrens' hospitals, and 13 at psychiatric hospitals (68). The increase in hospital-based clinics also increased training opportunities for child psychiatrists. A report by the Royal Medico-Psychological Association in 1960 indicated that there were then in Britain the equivalent of 16 full-time child psychiatrists and the equivalent of 16 full-time training posts (68). In order to reach their prescribed ratio of one child psychiatrist per 200,000 population, the RMPA recommended the establishment of 24 additional training posts to produce the 230 child psychiatrists they estimated would be needed by 1965.

Even though about 18% of the Maudsley graduates were going into child psychiatry, the number of child psychiatrists has not kept pace with the need. The RMPA estimate was actually inadequate (68). In Sweden, for example, the goal was one child psychiatric team per 50,000 population. Thus, when the reorganization of the Health Service places all psychiatric services for children under the Health Service in 1974 (59), the number of child psychiatrists will still be insufficient, and it has been recommended in some quarters that child psychiatric training be trebled (68).

At some clinics, treatment of children is combined with treatment of their parents. A longstanding program of this sort is the "Department of Parents and Children" at the Tavistock Clinic in London. More recently this approach has been broadened to encompass "Family Psychiatry," as at the Institute of Family Psychiatry of the Ipswich Hospital, under the direction of Dr. John Howells, a world leader in the "Family Psychiatry" movement (66, 69).

At any rate, it is expected that following the health service reorganization, the child (and family) psychiatric programs will be based at district general hospitals for the most part, and hopefully this move will bring to an end the pattern of fragmentation of services that has existed until now.

Two Special Problems

Drug Addiction

In the early part of this century, both Great Britain and the United States were faced with the problem of drug addiction. The magnitude of the problem was greater in the United States, which had an estimated addict population of about 782,000, compared to a much smaller number in Great Britain (32). Both countries passed similar laws to deal with the problem. In Britain the law was interpreted more liberally and passed into the hands of the medical profession, whereas the United States used a law enforcement approach.

During the 1960s, there was a significant rise in drug addiction in both countries. By 1968, Britain's heroin problem had reached its height; the addict population was doubling every six months, and the age range had dropped until 40% of the addicts were teenagers (93). At this time Parliament passed the Dangerous Drugs Act, and within one year Britain was the first nation in the western world to report a drop in the number of heroin addicts. Official statistics for 1970 revealed a decrease of 36 addicts, or a 2.4% reduction from a total of 1,466 registered for 1969 (6).

The Dangerous Drugs Regulations of 1968 established 14 drug treatment clinics at hospitals and other centers in London. Only licensed specialists, predominantly highly trained consultant psychiatrists, can prescribe heroin for addicts (41). All other doctors must report suspected addicts within seven days to the Home Office, which then refers them to one of the dispensing clinics operated by the Department of Health and Social Security. Only there can addicts receive a prescription for heroin. The 14 clinics in the London area handle about four-fifths of the nation's addicts (93). These clinics are usually attached to teaching hospitals, are financed out of general funds allocated by the National Health Service, and work closely with 40-50 voluntary agencies that are active in drug rehabilitation.

The British system of treating narcotic addicts is not simply a matter of doling out free heroin to all comers under the National Health Service auspices (6). One to three weeks of psychiatric interviews, case-history taking, and a definite commitment to therapy is involved. Addicts must report weekly to their clinic, where they must produce a urine sample for analysis. They are then given a prescription that can only be filled daily. This prevents them from selling supplies beyond their personal needs to other addicts. Each day's prescription comes with a sterile hypodermic needle and they inject the drug themselves. Recently, the use of methadone has increased, but British doctors use only minimum quantities (72, 93). They believe that this drug enables the addict to work and lead a somewhat normal life, even if he can't break the needle habit. If barbiturates or amphetamines are found in the addict's urine sample, however, doctors cut down on the dosage of methadone.

A clinic directed by Dr. Martin Mitcheson at University Hospital in London's Bloomsbury district has an "active list" of 100 addicts. There is also a staff of several part-time doctors, two full-time social workers, and a part-time nurse. In Great Britain, hospital clinics do not employ ex-addicts as paraprofessional aides (6). The clinic's unmarked building on Hampstead Road has recently undergone a $50,000 renovation and now has consulting offices, a carpeted waiting room, and poster-decorated meeting rooms. The treatment area consists of paneled cubicles for "shooting," oxygen tanks for overdose emergencies, and receptacles for used needles.

Actual rehabilitation of addicts, as opposed to containment of addiction and the crime it spawns, is still highly experimental. The heroin-maintenance clinics provide a frame, unrivaled elsewhere, for research into heroin addiction. Their clients are not merely a good sample but include almost all of the addicts in Britain. The records of addicts have been kept (the Home Office has kept an index of all known addicts for the past 50 years), and the addicts are known personally. Only recently, however, have British doctors begun to explore certain areas for research, such as what makes the difference between addicts and non-addicts from the same background and which treatment methods work best. For the past five years, clinic staffs have been learning how to prescribe to addicts, what psychiatric and social services are necessary, and what progress toward getting addicts off drugs is possible (72). Government guidelines permit each clinic consultant, as well as voluntary agencies, to determine the methods of treatment to be used in their own programs. Relations between these groups appear friendly and cooperative in contrast to the rivalry between such agencies in the United States.

The British believe they are doing something constructive about their drug problem. The police remain unarmed, and the streets are comparatively safe. The number of addicts sent to prison has fallen steadily since the 1968 law took effect. In addition, there is an improved work record among addicts in general. Forty percent of the addicts attending dispensing clinics are actually working, while only 20% had jobs when first admitted (77, 93).

The British theorize that supplying drugs to addicts undercuts any criminal profits and keeps organized crime out of the drug traffic. They have always considered addiction to be a medical rather than a moral problem.

There is a sharp contrast between Britain and the United States in the economics of addiction. It takes about $300 a week to support a habit in Washington, D.C., and almost nothing to support a habit in London. British addicts can be addicted to drugs without being addicted to crime to pay for them (93). Whether or not the British system would work in the United States is currently a controversial and political issue. There are differences between the two countries which must be considered. First, Great Britain is an island kingdom, much smaller than the United States, and protection against smugglers is easier. Secondly, the 560,000 estimated U.S. addict population represents a more profitable market for smugglers than the remaining 1,500 British addicts (77, 93). Finally, heroin has been banned in the United States for most of the twentieth century, while in Britain it has always been an acceptable drug for alleviating pain. This means that in the United States organized crime has had a long head start in developing its illegal distribution network.

Abortion

The Abortion Act of 1967 allows a doctor to terminate a pregnancy, if he and another doctor believe that continuation of the pregnancy would involve substantial risk to the physical or mental health of the pregnant woman or to the existing children in her family. In addition, a termination may be performed if there is a considerable risk that the child would be born seriously handicapped as a result of severe physical or mental abnormalities.

Before the 1967 Abortion Act, which went into effect in April 1968, few general practitioners referred patients to National Health Service gynecologists for abortion, unless the grounds were exceptional. Usually, general practitioners knew of doctors who would perform abortions upon the recommendation of a "sympathetic" psychiatric colleague (20). Thus, the burden of dealing with unwanted pregnancies was often placed on the psychiatrist, who had to justify the abortion on "mental grounds." Most psychiatrists resented this role, because it took them away from dealing with truly mentally ill patients and made them the scapegoat for society (27). In addition, many gynecologists would perform terminations under the title of "D. and C." for nurses, colleagues' daughters, and others who could arouse their sympathies (20). Thus, prior to 1968, if a woman wished to terminate an unwanted pregnancy, she had to find the "right" general practitioner or gynecologist; otherwise, her only recourse was to obtain an illegal abortion.

The 1967 Abortion Act requires that terminations be carried out in an approved hospital or nursing home, except in cases of immediate necessity, when the need for a second doctor is also dispensed with. Nursing homes must be approved annually by the Secretary of State, and at the end of 1968, 59 homes received approval. During the year, accredited nursing homes are inspected by medical and nursing officers of the Health Department. The Abortion Act also requires that the woman's age, marital status, duration of pregnancy, previous obstetric history, complications consequent to the abortion, and whether or not sterilization was performed, must be reported to the Chief Medical Officer of the Health and Social Security Department within seven days.

In the first year following the Abortion Act (April 27, 1968 to April 29, 1969), 38,000 abortions were performed in England and Wales (37). By 1970, the total number of terminations reached 80,723, and of these, 55% were carried out in National Health Service (N.H.S.) hospitals (38). An important consequence of the Abortion Act has been the redistribution of abortions among the categories of "N.H.S. therapeutic," "private therapeutic," and criminal. Prior to 1968, private therapeutic abortions were not recorded, and information on the number of criminal abortions could only be estimated from the number of hospital admissions following non-professional abortion attempts. Since 1966, the estimated increase in private abortions has been accompanied by a fall in hospital admissions for spontaneous and criminal abortions, which indicates that there was a transfer from the criminal to the legitimate sector. In 1968 there was a further shift from criminal abortions to N.H.S. therapeutic abortions. Finally, N.H.S. abortions have been increasing more rapidly than those done privately, but the overall rate of increase in terminations has been leveling off.

During the first year following the Abortion Act there was a death rate of 21 per 100,000 terminations compared with a maternal mortality rate of 24 per 100,000 total births (20). Thus, the initial claims that legal abortions would be dangerous have not been verified, although more information is needed on short- and long-term complications.

According to the Registrar's General Statistics for 1970, three-quarters of all legal abortions are undertaken on psychiatric grounds, but information on psychiatric aspects following termination is almost non-existent. In California, where abortion has been legal since November 1967, limited follow-up evaluations have revealed that few patients have developed severe post-abortal difficulty. True depression was rare, and suicide was almost absent (109). At least part of the emotional disturbance experienced by patients has been caused by the physical set-up of the clinical situation and the attitudes of staff and nursing personnel (80). In addition, the reaction to abortion is determined largely by the woman's previous psychological set.

Voluntary pregnancy advisory services have been established in London and Birmingham to assist women who are distressed by an unwanted pregnancy. By 1970, these organizations had seen over 7,800 women of whom 70% received therapeutic abortions. These voluntary services act as mediators between the people they serve and the administration of the medical health services, and they provide financial assistance to those in need. In Birmingham, where an abortion clinic operates closely with the Birmingham Pregnancy Advisory Service, the cost of a private abortion is about £65, and this figure is likely to decrease in the future.

Since the Abortion Act has been in effect, certain trends have become evident. There has been a shift from criminal and private therapeutic abortions to N.H.S. therapeutic abortions. Placing the decision of termination in the hands of the medical profession has reduced the delay between seeking abortion and its performance, when indicated. The medical profession has become more aware of the extent of despair and distress associated with an unwanted pregnancy and have been granting N.H.S. abortions on an increasing scale. Finally, the Abortion Act has brought about an increased interest in contraception and sterilization.

4

The psychiatrist and other mental health professionals

THE PSYCHIATRIST

At the end of 1970, there were approximately 2,800 psychiatrists in all grades in the National Health Service, a figure which represents almost all psychiatrists in the country. Most of them are in the Hospital Service, of whom 2,316 are in England. Of these 1,054 are consultants, and 267 are medical assistants. The remainder are in training positions (house officers, registrars, senior registrars). The consultant is the fully qualified specialist and the only one who may treat patients independently or make domiciliary visits. One hundred-twelve psychiatric consultants work with mental defectives, 169 with mentally ill children, and 773 with mentally ill adults (38).

Most of the consultants work in mental hospitals. Many carry some outpatient clinical responsibilities, and some are based in day hospitals. A number of consultants hold joint appointments; that is, in addition to their mental hospital post they may hold appointments with a general hospital psychiatric department, with a teaching hospital, with a local public health authority, or with some combination of these. There are few full-time teaching positions, but about 40 psychiatrists hold primary research positions with one of the nine psychiatric units of the Medical Research Council or elsewhere. There are about 150 part-time research appointments held by psychiatrists with primary responsibilities in other areas.

A number of psychiatrists hold administrative positions with the Health Service and elsewhere, but the position of "Medical Superintendent" of the mental hospital has been abolished. Mental hospitals, like other hospitals, are run by hospital management committees.

Most psychiatrists are employed full time in hospitals or on a joint appointment scheme, but a growing number have been going into part-time private practive. This entails reducing their Health Service commitment to a part-time arrangement. The most popular form this takes is called "maximum part-time," or 9/11 time. The full-time doctor is expected to give eleven half-days to the Health Service (5 1/2 days) per week. The "maximum part-time" arrangement allows the doctor two half-days for private practice. Most use this time for private diagnostic work, though some do psychotherapy or forensic psychiatry, etc. The part-time arrangement also enables the consultant to be paid for domiciliary visits from the very first, while the full-time doctor is not paid for the first eight visits in each quarter.

Psychiatrists in the Hospital Service, other than consultants, are not permitted private practice, nor to make domiciliary visits, nor even to take independent responsibility for treatment of patients within the hospital itself. The non-consultant posts are mainly training positions: senior house officer (the equivalent of assistant resident in the United States), registrar (resident), and senior registrar (advanced or senior resident). There are also even more junior posts equivalent to internship positions included in the total figures as "psychiatrists." A non-training category is "medical assistant," a sort of catch-all for registrars who did not obtain a senior registrar post, and for senior registrars who failed to get a consultant appointment. The registrar-senior registrar-consultant hierarchy is pyramidal, the number of consultant and senior registrar posts being strictly limited by the Health Ministry.

PROFESSIONAL ATTITUDES TOWARD PSYCHIATRY

The attitude of other medical specialists in Britain toward psychiatry is somewhat more skeptical and hostile than in the United States (79, 85). The attitude of the general practitioner is generally somewhat better but still rather negative. There are a number of probable reasons.

First, most older medical practitioners have had little or no training in psychiatry since, until fairly recently, the subject was not a usual part of the medical curriculum. In fact, some medical schools still have minimal provision for psychiatric teaching; even in 1970, six schools provided no clinical experience in the field. As recently as 1967, only 17 of the 22 medical schools in England and Wales had undergraduate chairs of psychiatry (67, 85). Second, until fairly recently the less capable physicians tended to drift into psychiatry. They often regarded the posts at isolated mental hospitals as a sinecure. The work was easy, and there was much free time to take advantage of the golf, fishing, and other out-door activities available in the countryside surrounding the institution. Consequently, to opt for this specialty has often been regarded as a confession of incompetence, laziness, or both. Third, the isolation from the majority of physicians, seemingly imposed by the remoteness of the mental hospitals, has continued even after much psychiatric activity has moved into the community. General hospital psychiatric units, for example, are still physically separated from the rest of the hospital wards, usually in their own buildings (often converted poor law work house units) on the hospital grounds. The psychiatric staff tend to remain apart from the main stream of hospital activity, and interaction with other specialists is generally confined to consultation about particular problems and patients. Finally, there is the aura of magic, fear of the unknown, and anxiety over personal difficulties which stigmatize psychiatry in the eye of the general public, a stigma to which the physician is not immune.

On the other hand, the psychiatrists' position *vis-à-vis* other doctors has much improved since the advent of the Health Service. Their basic pay scale is the same as that of other specialists, though bonuses may be less frequent; and their status, while still definitely below most other specialities, has risen somewhat. Their position is similar to that of a minority group whose living conditions have not yet reached those of their neighbors but who are no longer overtly oppressed.

Although some psychiatrists have had the initiative to bring their profession closer to the other medical fields, for the most part they have remained aloof from their confreres and have thus perpetuated their own isolation. Some seem to reflect a sense of inferiority or second-class citizenship. Some choose to ignore or deny the situation, pointing to the heavily organic and physical orientation of the British psychiatrist as evidence of his basic identification with his medical colleagues.

For the most part, however, psychiatrists express resentment at their status, which they regard as discriminatory. They point out, for example, that merit awards, particularly in the higher categories, are received less frequently by psychiatrists than by other specialists.

The psychoanalytic movement is weak in Britain, and there is only a handful of analysts, some of whom are not even physicians. In general, Freudian psychology does not enjoy a high reputation among British psychiatrists. Most psychiatrists have had little training in psychoanalytic theory or dynamic psychotherapy and hence tend to attack it as alien. Some take the position that Freudian ideas are all right in their place, but that British psychiatrists do not have the time needed to employ these methods. They point out that they are confronted by large numbers of patients for whom they must provide symptomatic relief. They tend, however, to refer patients who might benefit from psychotherapy and who in the United States would be treated by a psychiatrist, to social workers, ostensibly for "case work"; consequently, much of the psychotherapy that is carried out is, in fact, done by the psychiatric social workers, who are more psychodynamically oriented than the psychiatrists.

A psychoanalytic bastion in the medical community is the Tavistock Centre, whose high standards have contributed significantly to the maintenance of a positive image of psychoanalysis. Even this outstanding institution, which receives financial support from the Health Service, is held in greater esteem by social workers than by physicians, including psychiatrists.

Bickering between analytic groups with different ideas and philosophies has not helped the situation, nor has the ready provision of psychoanalytic training to non-medical people endeared the field to those seeking to defend psychiatry's medical identity.

A number of British psychiatrists are vociferously anti-psychoanalytic and frequently speak out in blatantly defensive articles in the various journals against psychoanalysis and all that it represents. Particularly prominent in this group are the writings of William Sargent and Hans J. Eysenck. Some espouse a conciliatory approach between psychoanalytic and behavioristic ideas. The Maudsley, which trains most of the teachers of psychiatry in Britain, has consistently maintained a traditional organic-physiological orientation. Probably the most psychodynamically oriented psychiatrists in Britain are child psychiatrists who tend to use the psychoanalytic model of psycho-sexual development in their work with children. Their number, however, is relatively small.

ORGANIZED PSYCHIATRY

Organized medicine had its start in Britain with the formation in 1518 of the College of Physicians of London (67). This group, organized after the fashion of the guilds, was created to protect the legitimate interests of physicians and evolved into the present Royal College of Physicians. (By history and common usage the term "college" came to be applied to the highest professional bodies in medicine which had special responsibilities, functions, and standards. The term "Royal College" is used when the organization has been granted a Royal Charter giving it status and official recognition as the established spokesman and advisory body to the government with respect to the particular field.)

The first professional organization of psychiatrists in Britain (and, it is claimed, in the world) was the Association of Medical Officers of Hospitals for the Insane, formed in 1841. The name of the organization was changed in 1865 to the Medico-Psychological Association of Great Britain and Ireland. The Association was granted a Royal Charter in 1926 and renamed the Royal Medico-Psychological Association (RMPA).

This organization became the dominant professional standard-bearer for British psychiatry. It brought psychiatrists together for discussion of their common problems, served to transmit information on developments in the field through its official publication, *The British Journal of Psychiatry,* and concerned itself with standards of psychiatric practice and education (94, 95, 96, 97, 98). Despite its Royal Charter, many matters of close concern to psychiatrists were the responsibility, not of the RMPA, but of the Royal College of Physicians.

For example, because it was not a Royal College, the RMPA was not an official spokesman for psychiatry either with the government or in the higher councils of medicine. This task fell to the Royal College of Physicians (RCP). Membership in the Royal College of Physicians is by "membership examination" and is a necessary prerequisite for advancement in the Health Service. Yet many psychiatrists were, in effect, denied a membership examination, as they considered it unreasonable to have their competence in psychiatry assessed by an examination in another discipline. Although the membership of the Royal College of Physicians did, in fact, include a number of psychiatrists, the RCP could not be considered an adequate spokesman for psychiatric affairs, because of the lower status enjoyed by psychiatry in relation to other specialties, and the still strained relationships in some quarters between psychiatrists and other physicians.

While a number of psychiatrists were satisfied with the *status quo,* many others felt the need for a Royal College independent of the Royal College of Physicians in order to reach the higher councils of medicine and to be in a position to speak for themselves and control their own standards of practice.

It has been the history of the various specialties that they have sought to form their own particular Royal Colleges. Thus, the Royal College of Surgeons was granted its charter in 1800; the Royal College of Obstetrics and Gynecology received its charter in 1936; and the Royal College of Pathology was estabished in 1970.

Discussion of the possibility of establishing a Royal College of Psychiatrists had taken place within the RMPA from time to time almost from its very inception in 1926, but it was not until the early 1960s that this move gained momentum (15, 19, 89).

Abetting this movement within the RMPA was another organization called the Society of Clinical Psychiatrists, a group of senior psychiatrists who function in a fashion analogous to that of the Group for the Advancement of Psychiatry in the United States (67). Resistance to the movement came from some of the RMPA establishment. The younger psychiatrists in particular were dissatisfied that the examination in psychiatry was controlled not by psychiatrists, but by physicians in other disciplines. Representations to the government in behalf of psychiatry had to be made by the Royal College of Physicians, who also nominated the psychiatric advisors to government committees and commissions. The psychiatrists had no direct representation on the Joint Consultants Committee, nor on the Joint Medical Council (67). They resented particularly their lack of representation on the Merit Awards Committee, pointing out that only 14% of psychiatrists received merit awards in 1962, in contrast to over 50% in medicine and surgery; this, despite the fact that 40% of the hospital beds were occupied by psychiatric patients.

The Royal College of Psychiatrists was finally granted its charter by the Queen on April 30, 1971, after a ten-year struggle. With the grant of the charter the Royal Medico-Psychological Association became the Royal College of Psychiatrists.

Categories of membership in the new Royal College follow the pattern of the old guilds; i.e., Fellow (Master), Member (Journeyman), and Inceptor (Apprentice). The latter category is unique in that it provides for trainee members. Members use the initials MRCPsych. following their names; Fellows, FRCPsych.

It is difficult to predict the effect which the Royal College will have on the future course of psychiatric development. Its stated aims include the maintenance of high standards in the practice of psychiatry, and among its first orders of business is the establishment of a "higher examination" in psychiatry. There will be one national examination which will regulate national standards and will signify the successful completion of a prescribed period of training. In addition, the Royal College looks forward to its role as a consultative body in relation to matters of public and professional interest concerning psychiatry. It will have a direct place on the Joint Consultants Committee and will thus have a voice together with the other Royal Colleges in advising the government in professional matters. The Royal College will nominate representatives to the Central Health Service Council, the General Nursing Council, and the Central Committee for Postgraduate Medical Education. It has already acquired a place on the Merit Awards Committee and hopes to bring about a more equitable distribution of awards (67). Among its other goals are the promotion of improved methods of prevention and treatment and the encouragement of research.

EDUCATION OF THE PSYCHIATRIST

Medical education in Britain is conducted in "teaching hospitals" which are affiliated with one or another of the 17 universities granting medical degrees. In London there are 12 teaching hospitals which serve as undergraduate medical schools, as well as centers for postgraduate training, and 14 others providing postgraduate education only. All are linked with the University of London. In addition, there are nine teaching hospital-medical schools in other parts of England and one in Wales, which provide both undergraduate and graduate education in medicine.

Students generally enter medical school at age 18, after completing high school. The medical diploma, awarded after six years of study, usually confers the degree of Bachelor of Medicine. A year of internship (called junior house officer) is required for registration. The degrees of Doctor of Medicine (MD) or Master of Surgery (MS) are considered advanced degrees, conferred by the university after completion of additional study and clinical work. Membership or fellowship in one of the Royal Colleges, (MRCP, FRCP, FRCS), usually a prerequisite for advancement, is also looked upon as the attainment of an advanced degree, as are the special diplomas issued following training in a specialty, such as the Diploma in Psychological Medicine (DPM). Hence, the British doctor tends to have more initials following his name than does his American counterpart.

Undergraduate Training

Undergraduate medical education is conducted in two stages. The first is a pre-clinical period of five or six terms (2 1/2 to 3 years). The first pre-clinical year is really a pre-medical year; the second and third pre-clinical years are concerned with anatomy, physiology, and chemistry and may also include pathology, microbiology, and pharmacology (called "paraclinical subjects") (117, 118). The second stage is the three-year clinical period. If the paraclinical subjects have not been included in the pre-clinical years, they are included in the clinical period. Clinical teaching consists of varying amounts of seminar or lecture time and a varying amount of time spent in clinical clerkships on the wards. Students are assigned to medical "firms" (services) for periods of one to three months in the various specialties.

Students on a psychiatry firm are taught bedside clerking, presentation of case histories, and outpatient clerking. They attend seminars, and are tutored individually by members of the staff. In addition, the students visit psychiatric and subnormality hospitals, social service or drug clinics, and may accompany a consultant on a domiciliary visit. They may be taught the principles of psychotherapy, often without doing any of it. In some centers one-way screens or closed circuit television are used to allow unobtrusive observation of psychotherapy in progress. Occasionally students conduct some psychotherapy under close supervision.

The length of time set aside for seminar teaching of psychiatry in the clinical years varics between 0-89 hours, with a mean of 30 hours. Lecture time spent in psychiatry in the various universities during the clinical years ranges between 6-39 hours. In 1970 six of the medical schools had no clinical clerkship in psychiatry whatsoever. In the others there was a range of from 36-468 hours of clinical time spent on the wards.

Postgraduate Training in Psychiatry

Postgraduate training in psychiatry is conducted at a number of training centers around the country (107). There are 157 mental hospitals recognized for training for the DPM, 47 general hospitals and 29 university training centers. The largest of these is the Maudsley Institute of Psychiatry, a part of the University of London.

Following completion of medical school studies, there is a one-year internship (called the pre-registration year). The student then serves as senior house officer for one year. This assignment is similar to the assistant-resident level in the United States. Service is chiefly with a firm in the speciality for which he seeks training. He then obtains a post as a registrar which he holds for two years while trying to find a senior registrar post. If he is unable to get such a position, he may become a "medical assistant" in a mental hospital. There are in fact many more doctors in hospital posts than can ever hope to become consultants because of the limited number of consultant positions. Those who do obtain senior registrar appointments get highly variable training, although they usually receive a wide range of experience. Most posts are intended to provide service rather than training. A number of senior registrars fail to find posts as consultants, and they, too, may be forced to accept medical-assistant positions.

The "medical assistant" grade came in following the Platt Report (54) in 1961. It was intended to provide permanent appointments for doctors with several years of service unable to get consultant positions after their period of training. It was also thought to be suitable for part-time employment of experienced general practitioners with visiting hospital appointments.

However, the grade has not been popular, because of its name and the idea of "assistantship," that is, the restriction that the medical assistant may not treat cases except under the supervision of the consultant. It has been recommended that the name be changed to "hospital specialist," and that the holder of the post have freedom to treat patients independently while having available advice from consultants as needed. Although the British Medical Association wanted more consultant posts, with a strong career ladder leading from registrar to consultant, the Health Department decided instead to reduce the number of registrar posts.

Recognition of successful completion of postgraduate psychiatric education is bestowed by the Diploma in Psychological Medicine (DPM). The standard requirement for the DPM is two years experience in a recognized psychiatric hospital and a stipulated amount of general experience in medicine and neurology. Several of the university departments, including the Maudsley, offer their own DPM examinations. Other university departments collaborate with mental hospitals in their regions to instruct registrars preparing for the Conjoint Board Diploma. The Conjoint Board is set up by the various universities to offer examinations that are uniform throughout the country, in contrast to those offered by the individual university training centers bestowing the DPM. Outside of London there are only two to three students per year preparing for university diplomas. Most others prepare for the Conjoint Board Examinations, which apparently are somewhat less difficult.

Evaluation of Psychiatric Education

The first comprehensive review of medical education in Britain was made in 1942-44 by the Goodenough Committee whose report "deplored the low standard of existing diplomas in psychological medicine" and advocated better preparation for future psychiatrists. While they acknowledged that postgraduate psychiatric training would inevitably continue to be given in a number of mental hospitals scattered throughout the country, they urged that two additional national teaching centers be established, where much higher standards of training would be maintained.

More recently the status of medical education was re-studied by the Royal Commission on Medical Education (57). A special task force of the Royal Commission headed by Dr. G. M. Carstairs (13) undertook a survey of psychiatric education and training. Although they found the picture in 1968 "not as black" as in 1944, they felt there is still much to be desired.

Many psychiatric teachers in Britain are still dissatisfied with the amount of time in the curriculum devoted to psychology, sociology, and related subjects. They believe that if students are to develop an understanding of human behavior and be able to recognize the importance of emotional and social factors when treating patients, their education in these topics should start early. The survey of medical school curricula conducted by Carstairs showed that only one or two medical schools taught substantial courses in the behavioral sciences, while many provided only a short series of lectures to students during their pre-clinical training. Although the situation has improved to a certain extent, the amount of time devoted to these studies is still quite low. Which aspects and what amount of sociology and psychology, and who should teach them (clinicians vs. psychologists and sociologists), are currently being debated.

The Carstairs report considers that the chief improvements have been the development of a major postgraduate program based at the Maudsley Hospital in London and the creation of new academic departments of psychiatry in all the provincial medical schools, as well as in some of the London medical schools. However, several of the London medical schools still had no chair in psychiatry. The first chair in psychiatry at Oxford was established only in 1968.

By 1964-65 the Maudsley Institute of Psychiatry was training 174 doctors, some of whom were preparing for the University of London Diploma in Psychological Medicine (now replaced by a Master of Philosophy degree), while others were preparing for the DPM examinations offered by the Conjoint Board. The Institute of Psychiatry has played a major role in training teachers and research workers over the past 20 years and probably will continue in that role.

A new medical school at Nottingham University, which opened in 1970, has set aside 120 psychiatric beds for the use of students and the medical school. They have placed more emphasis on psychiatry than most medical schools in Britain generally do. Community medicine and psychiatry are introduced during the pre-clinical years.

The Royal Medico-Psychological Association, prior to becoming the "Royal College of Psychiatrists," conducted a survey (95) which showed that between one-fourth and one-half of the hospitals recognized as suitable for training leading to the Conjoint Board Diploma in Psychological Medicine did not meet the minimum requirements set down for such training. The following data are based upon their survey, to which the vast majority of approved training centers responded.

Of the established minimal criteria for approved programs, the only ones met by all training centers were that all have at least two approved psychiatric consultants in addition to consultants in other branches of medicine, and that all have formal liaison with a general hospital and with a psychiatric outpatient department. Of the 148 mental hospitals responding to the survey, 27% had no psychologists, 20% did not conduct regular clinical case conferences, 22% did not have adequate library facilities, 45% had no clinical tutor (i.e., a consultant specifically designated to carry out instruction of registrars), 36% had no training in group psychotherapy, and 50% had no training in individual psychotherapy. Seventy percent had no consultant-conducted seminars on psychotherapy. Seventy percent of the hospital programs had no Journal

Club. Eighty percent had no instruction in mental subnormality, and 86% had no outpatient experience in this field. Thirty-six percent had no training or experience in community psychiatry.

Of the 42 responding general hospital units approved for DPM training, 60% had no psychologist, and 38% had an inadequate medical library from the standpoint of psychiatric books and journals. Even 16% of the 26 teaching hospitals which responded to the survey had an inadequate medical library as far as psychiatric volumes and journals were concerned.

Forty-two percent of all psychiatric training centers have training in neurology by lecture and outpatient clinics only, and 36% by case conference only.

As a consequence of these studies of medical and psychiatric education, a general upgrading of both may be expected. It should be emphasized, however, that on the whole the British psychiatrist is as well prepared for the performance of his duties as the average American psychiatrist is for his (75). The many unique and ingenious programs developed in Britain could not have been possible were it not for many outstanding, dedicated, and well-prepared people.

EDUCATION IN THE ALLIED PROFESSIONS

State registers have been established for nurses, dieticians, occupational therapists, laboratory technicians, etc., which specify the minimum training required to qualify for registration in the particular profession. Only state-registered members may be employed in the National Health Service. Among those professions related to mental health, only psychology does not have such a standard educational and registration requirement.

Nursing

Usually three years of hospital training are required to qualify for registration in nursing. Whereas in the United States nurses' training is generic with the later option to specialize, in Britain training for each of the three categories of registered nurse is separate and distinct. These categories are: State Registered Nurse (SRN) to designate the general nurse; Registered Sick Children's Nurse (RSCN); and Registered Mental Nurse (RMN). In the latter category, there is even the specialized Registered Nurse for the Mentally Subnormal (RNMS). Registration in one category does not qualify for practice in another. Of course it is possible for registered nurses already trained in one category to take additional training in another, and in fact, this is often done.

While not nearly as common as in the United States, there are a number of schools offering degree courses which combine nurses' training with the study of related subjects like psychology, sociology, and biology. Several hospitals offer two-year SRN courses for those who have already graduated in other subjects. It is also possible to combine nurses' training with training in social and preventive medicine.

The British equivalent of the practical nurse in the United States is the "State Enrolled Nurse" (SEN), training for which consists of a two-year hospital course emphasizing practical work. The SEN may work in hospitals under the supervision of registered nurses.

Social Work

For a long time, training in social work in Britain was haphazard and chaotic. A handful of social workers had university training. Most other people working in the field, and called "social workers," had little or no training.

As recently as 1965, the London *Times* reported that there were only 300 fully-qualified psychiatric social workers in Great Britain. For certification, a university degree was required, followed by field experience and a postgraduate year of psychiatric social work training in a special university center at London, Manchester, or Edinburgh. Most so-called psychiatric social workers were uncertified, having had various degrees of training or experience. A number of people working in mental hospitals as psychiatric social workers were in fact trained as mental nurses. Others had had some courses in social studies, and yet others, no formal training.

In 1959 a study of social work training and the need for social workers in Britain was conducted under the leadership of Dame Eileen Younghusband. The recommendations of the "Younghusband Report" (120), which aimed at improving the quality and quantity of social work training, led to the enactment of the Heath Visiting and Social Work (Training) Act of 1962, which established the Council for Training in Social Work to upgrade social work education. As a consequence, there were two types of social-work training in addition to the university training program.

Previously, certification was a specialized one in the particular area of social work in which the person had been trained. In addition to psychiatric social work, certification was available in medical social work, child welfare, probation, and welfare work. Fully-trained certified psychiatric social workers enjoyed high social status, although they were poorly paid.

For medical social workers and psychiatric social workers a university degree, diploma, or certificate course in social science was taken, followed by a university course in applied social studies, or by specialized training for a particular service organized by the profession concerned. Alternatively, a full-time, two-year course at a college of further education could be taken leading to the Certificate in Social Work of the Council for Training in Social Work. Under a temporary scheme to increase the number of trained workers, the certificate could be obtained by completing a special one-year course open to mature students with suitable experience.

An additional program that followed upon the Younghusband Report, intended to supplement the courses offered by the universities and technical colleges, established the National Institute for Social Work Training, both to train experienced social workers to teach their profession and to provide advanced refresher courses, in addition to carrying out other functions related to training and research.

Recent years have seen a significant increase in the number of social workers employed by the local authorities. The Health Service had frozen the salary scales for those employed in hospitals but not for those employed by local authorities. Consequently, by upgrading salaries, local authorities generally outbid the hospitals (including the mental hospitals) for the services of the available social workers, particularly the most qualified ones. At the end of 1963, there were 2,175 social workers employed by the Local Authority Health and Welfare services in various capacities (51). Of these, 215 were certified, and 53 held the Certificate of Social Work. By the end of 1970, there were 5,476 social workers to be found in the Local Authority Health and Welfare services (including 175 employed by voluntary organizations as agents of local authority). Of these, 414 were fully qualified, and 1,077 held a certificate in social work. In the Local Authority Mental Health services at the end of 1970, there were 207 fully-qualified psychiatric social workers, 447 holding the certificate, and 1,284 partially trained or untrained workers (38).

In 1968, an intensive study of the Local Authority Social Services in England and Wales was undertaken by a commission, headed by Fredrick Seebohm (101). As a consequence of the Seebohm Report, a major reorganization of the Local Authority Social Services began in January 1971. Social workers from the local-authority Children's Department, Welfare Department, and Mental Health Section of the Health Department were brought together under a single agency called the Local Authority Social Service Department. This department now assumes responsibility for all mental health functions which were formerly under the administrative supervision of the Medical Officer of Health. Under this scheme the social workers no longer function in their specialized roles (i.e., child care worker, welfare worker, or psychiatric social worker), but rather all function as "generic social workers." The psychiatric social workers, who had constituted a small elite core of usually better-trained workers, were greatly outnumbered by the workers from the other two areas. As a result of implementing the Seebohm Report, the local authority programs related to mental health have undergone a significant change, and the quality of service during the reorganization has, it is hoped, only temporarily fallen. Further changes can be expected when the Redcliffe-Maud Report on Local Government Reorganization is put into effect (58).

The Seebohm Report leads social-work training in the direction of providing generic case workers rather than workers with specialized training (1, 33, 101). High priority is given to the further training of field-work teachers and training officers. The generic training program seeks to equip students to work with individuals, groups, or communities on problems of all sorts. Training in social planning and administrative structure is provided. Advanced courses, above the basic professional level, are necessary in particular fields of knowledge and practice, such as delinquency and mental health, in specific social work methods, and for work in particular settings such as residential homes and schools.

Psychology

There are no standardized requirements for training in psychology in the Health Service. Most psychologists are educational psychologists who work for the Education Department rather than the Health Service. They are largely responsible for working with emotionally disturbed children. Their education begins with an undergraduate degree in psychology, following which they may obtain three years of teaching or equivalent experience with children, after which a one-year university course is taken; or, alternatively, they may go on immediately after completing their undergraduate degree to take a three-year university course, of which the first two years are spent as classroom teachers along with some simultaneous course work, followed by a full-time education year similar to the one-year course noted above.

Clinical psychology is a much less well-known discipline in England than in the United States. Following completion of an undergraduate degree in psychology, a two-year course which includes clinical assignments is taken. Alternatively, a four-year course leading to a higher degree may be pursued. Until recently the handful of clinical psychologists in Britain were to be found only in the mental hospitals.

RESEARCH IN PSYCHIATRY

Since 1920, the promotion of medical research has been the responsibility of the Medical Research Council, an autonomous body maintained by the government (34). The Council is assisted by three Advisory Boards in the areas of clinical research, biological research, and tropical medicine research. The Council supports and subsidizes medical research in three major ways. Primarily, it operates a number of its own research units ranging from the major National Institute for Medical Research in London to over 70 small units attached to universities and hospitals around the country. In addition, the Council awards project grants to independent workers, based mainly at universities and hospitals, and a number of fellowships and scholarships for research training.

There are nine research units specifically identified as psychiatric which are operated by the Medical Research Council, but a number of others have psychiatric implications. Among the relevant projects are the Applied Psychology Research Unit at Cambridge; the Brain Metabolism Unit at Edinburgh; the Unit for Reserach on the Chemical Pathology of Mental Disorders in Sheffield; a Clinical Psychiatry Research Unit at Graylingwell, Chichester; a Unit for the Study of Environmental Factors in Mental and Physical Illness at the London School of Economics; a Unit for Research on Epidemiology of Psychiatric Illness at Edinburgh; a Unit for Research on the Neural Mechanisms of Behavior at the University College, London; a Neuroendocrinology Unit at Oxford; a Neuropharmacology Unit at Birmingham; a Neuropsychiatric Research Unit at the Medical Research Council Laboratories at Surrey; and the two units located at the Maudsley Institute of Psychiatry: the Psychiatric Genetics Research Unit and the Social Psychiatry Research Unit.

THE BRITISH PSYCHIATRIST—PROSPECTS FOR THE FUTURE

It seems likely that the general upgrading of psychiatric education at both undergraduate and graduate levels, which may be expected to result from the implementation of the Todd Report (57) and the efforts of the Royal College of Psychiatrists, comes at a time when psychiatrists will be having a narrowing role. The anticipated alteration in the organization of local-authority services as a consequence of the Redcliffe-Maud Report (58), as well as the significant changes in the organization of the National Health Service heralded by the Ministry of Health's White Paper (59), are both bound to weaken the position of the MOH, and hence of the physician generally in the local-authority service systems. The Seebohm Report has placed most community .psychiatric services in the hands of the new unified Social Service Department, to which psychiatrists are mere advisors (101).

These changes of organization suggest that the psychiatrist will become even more firmly implanted in the hospital service rather than increase his activity in local-authority-based community programs. With the run-down of the mental hospitals and the projected continuing emphasis on the development of psychiatric units in district general hospitals, however, the psychiatrist will be moving from the mental hospital to the community general hospital (42).

It is likely that his work here will focus primarily upon the treatment of psychiatric emergencies and rapid treatment and early discharge after brief hospitalization of mentally ill patients, who will tend to come for treatment earlier in the course of their illness. The psychiatrists will probably have little or nothing to do with the elderly "psychogeratric" patient, and will become further removed from the chronically ill, whose rehabilitation in the community will be dealt with mainly by the social workers.

Thus, it seems that in the future (at least for the next five years) British psychiatry will become concerned more with acute than with chronic problems, will be based increasingly at general hospitals rather than mental hospitals, will make more effective use of existing personnel, but will not show significant increases in numbers of trained specialists. The new graduates, however, will be of overall higher quality than in the past and will press to bring the psychiatrists into closer relationship with the patient being treated. Continuity of care thus will remain difficult to achieve as it relates to the chronically ill adult but will be easier in acute situations. Prevention of chronic illness will also become a major objective.

It is unlikely that the general practitioner will become more involved in the problems of mental illness than he has been in the past. The overall status of the psychiatrist and his relationship with his other medical colleagues, however, will most probably improve.

5

The providers of the mental health service

THE HOSPITAL SERVICES

Mental Hospitals

There are approximately 150 mental hospitals in England and Wales, ranging in size from fewer than 100 beds to several thousand. When the National Health Service was put into effect in 1948, all of the nation's mental institutions were incorporated within the hospital services. The major aim of the Mental Health Act of 1959 was to establish the treatment of mental disorder on the same basis as that for other kinds of illnesses. Provisions were made for voluntary admissions, and the use of compulsory powers was curtailed (83). Procedural safeguards to protect the patient from unnecessary detention were established, calling for a mental health review Tribunal, appointed by the Lord Chancellor, for each of the 14 hospital regions. At the end of 1970, fewer than 7% of the resident mental patients were compulsorily detained (38, 44). Most hospitals are quite large, built in Victorian times in outlying areas, and intended to provide custodial care.

The shift in emphasis in the hospitals from custodial care to a therapeutic orientation was initially seen largely in terms of the administration of physical treatments such as electroshock, insulin, and later the tranquilizer drugs. The emphasis on rehabilitation of chronic, apathetic, isolated patients resulted in the introduction of other approaches, beginning with the "open door" and therapeutic community and leading to the establishment of rehabilitation wards and industrial therapy programs.

Even within the hospitals there was wide variation in the degree of emphasis placed upon these rehabilitative efforts. Some hospitals reorganized themselves significantly in order to emphasize the new community orientation. Others, however, retained almost intact their traditional approaches and organization. A peculiar illustration of this is to be found at Littlemore Hospital in Oxford, where one half of the hospital continues to be organized along traditional lines while the other half has made major reorganizational changes.

The introduction of industrial therapy programs into the rehabilitative effort was intended to give the patients productive work more closely resembling actual industrial conditions than the occupational therapy activities formerly utilized. By means of contracts with local industry, particular projects were assigned to patients for which they were paid small sums. Often the regimen resembled that in an actual factory, with punching in and out on time clocks, repeated assessment of work performance, with wage increases reflecting improvement, etc. In some instances the hospital industrial therapy program became an actual industry. At Graylingwell Hospital in Chichester, the hospital workshops provide the sterilized bandages and other supplies for all of the hospitals in the district; while the Cheadle Royal Hospital has become a major commercial production service, called Cheadle Royal Industries Ltd., where a hospital factory makes and markets a variety of items.

The programs at Littlemore, Graylingwell, and Mapperley in Nottingham illustrate the approaches developed by the hospital, largely based on extension of hospital services into the community. These programs vary in the intensity of collaboration with the local authority services.

General Hospitals

The development of psychiatric services in general hospitals has had its major proliferation in the Manchester area. By 1948 the Manchester Regional Hospital Board had already decided to utilize the district general hospitals as the base for psychiatric treatment. The poor-law units of the community general hospitals were abolished, and the buildings were converted to psychiatric units for their adjacent general hospitals. Within each group of hospitals governed by a Hospital Management Committee responsible to the Manchester Regional Hospital Board, there has tended to be at least one general hospital with psychiatric beds.

The trend has been to carry out all inpatient psychiatric treatment within the general hospital setting rather than in the traditional mental hospitals. Inpatient services were augmented by extensive day-hospital provisions. This tended to move psychiatric services into community settings earlier in the Manchester region than elsewhere, and resulted in shorter lengths of patient stay in the general hospitals than had been the experience within the traditional mental hospitals. By 1960, when the ratio of psychiatric beds per thousand population in England and Wales was 3.3, the Manchester ratio had already been reduced to 2.7 per thousand (106). Despite the Manchester experience, there has been only a small increase in the number of general hospital units in England and Wales. In 1960 there were 82 such units, and by 1968 the number has risen only to 88, although the Hospital Plan called for 168 such units to be in operation by 1975 (91). It is expected that the development of general-hospital psychiatric units will be greatly accelerated in the future.

The Queen's Park Hospital in Blackburn is illustrative of the large general hospital inpatient unit which has completely eliminated the need for mental hospital beds, by providing day hospital and other services developed by the psychiatric facility. The program at Salford illustrates the combined efforts of general hospital and local authority services to provide community facilities for the psychiatric patients. Although this service continues to utilize the mental hospital for some of its patients, its goal is ultimately to care for all of the region's psychiatric inpatients in the general hospital's psychiatric beds.

The program at St. Mary Abbots illustrates the function of a general hospital psychiatric service within a London borough, where again the emphasis is on treating all comers. Here, too, a sizeable day-hospital program and active outpatient service augment the relatively small inpatient unit.

This emphasis upon providing total care for all inpatients, chronic as well as acute, is more characteristic of general hospital psychiatric services in Britain than in the United States. In Britain those in charge of the traditional mental hospitals have been concerned that development of general hospital psychiatric services would tend to "cream off" the more responsive patients and would relegate the unrewarding chronic long-stay patients to the mental hospital (83). In order to combat this idea the general hospitals have stressed their ability to handle the whole problem and hence eliminate the need for the mental institution altogether. In 1971 the Health Ministry recommended a gradual phasing out of mental institutions with the complete transfer of inpatient psychaitric treatment to general hospital psychiatric units (42). It is anticipated that community facilities will be developed to provide other necessary services, such as day centers, sheltered workshops, outpatient clinics, work therapy programs, halfway houses, etc.

While the general hospital units actually do provide a certain degree of liaison between psychiatrists and specialists in other fields, psychiatric services still tend to be separated from those offered other general hospital patients. Often the psychiatric unit is in a separate building, not an integral part of the general hospital proper. Communication between psychiatrists and other specialists is not great, and a certain attitude of suspicion of psychiatric patients tends to remain in many general hospitals. Very few general hospital psychiatric units have been built for that purpose; consequently, their facilities are often as ill-suited for psychiatric treatment as are the facilities in traditional mental hospitals. Indeed, in the case of the larger (over 100 beds) general hospital units, the effect is sometimes that of a mental hospital housed on the general hospital campus.

Teaching Hospitals

Teaching hospitals have remained for the most part outside of the community mental health orbit, just as they have remained outside of the jurisdiction of the Regional Hospital Boards. The psychiatric services of the teaching hospitals draw their patients from all over Britain on the basis of their interest for teaching purposes. The educational emphasis has tended to minimize the interest in providing service to the community. Consequently, teaching hospitals have remained aloof from developments towards providing community mental health services. A single notable exception is the Maudsley Hospital, which has undertaken to serve the Borough of Camberwell, in which it is located, as a catchment area. The Maudsley, however, is in many respects unique among psychiatric teaching hospitals.

LOCAL AUTHORITY SERVICES

When the National Health Service was set up in 1948, its tripartite structure retained the local authorities' responsibility for providing public health services and specifically, preventive services and care and aftercare for the sick. The Mental Health Act of 1959, which emphasized the shift from institutional to community care for the mentally disordered, spelled out ways in which the statutory responsibilities of the local authority for providing preventive and aftercare services was to be applied in the case of the mentally ill and subnormal. These provisions include sheltered living accommodations, such as hostels, for those unable to return to completely independent community life, or for those who had no families to return to upon discharge from the hospital; sheltered workshops or occupational centers operated as transition services to permit the return to industrial work, or on a continuing basis for those unable to assume the responsibilities of regular employment; and day centers or social clubs to permit the resocialization of those returned to the community after many years of social isolation in mental hospitals (17). Additionally, other services, such as ambulances to transport people to day hospitals, are part of the local-authority responsibility. It is not an exaggeration to say that the response by the local authorities was less than enthusiastic, and the implementation of these responsibilities, while extremely varied, has remained on the meager side.*

By the end of 1970, only 85,682 mentally ill persons (including 620 children) were receiving mental health services provided by local authorities in England. Of these 2,755 were receiving residential care. Twenty new hostels were built during the year, providing 371 places. There were 1,938 social workers in the local-authority mental health services, of whom 207 were fully qualified and 477 held the Certificate in Social Work (38).

The projections of the local authorities anticipated 563 fully qualified social workers in their health and welfare services by 1968. As late as 1970 there were fewer than 400. Some local authorities tend to have large numbers of social workers, many of whom are fully qualified, while other local authorities have few or none.

Casework and psychotherapy are also often provided by the social work staff, usually under the "supervision" of a psychiatric consultant from a nearby mental or general hospital who holds a part-time joint appointment with the local authority. Most local authority services for the mentally ill serve those who were discharged from mental hospitals; that is, they are rehabilitative rather than preventive.

In a few instances, the local authority took the initiative in developing community services for the mentally disordered. Such programs were the product of an enterprising far-seeing Medical Officer of Health combined with the support of the local government council in providing funds for these purposes. The funds are required, not only for the construction of facilities, but for the employment of staff, such as social workers. Each program is a unique reflection of the ingenuity of its creator. A fine example of such a program was found in the London Borough of Camden to be described later. One of the most outstanding examples of a comprehensive local authority service is that of the London Borough of Newham.

In a few local authorities, as noted earlier, psychiatric services for

*See the article by J. Roper, "Group attacks inadequate care for the mentally ill," London *Times*, October 24, 1973, p. 1.

children include child guidance. Some guidance clinics were encompassed within the mental health section of the Health Department, but this was the exception rather than the rule. For the most part, services for children have been fragmented and separate from the regular mental health programs.

While the Health Ministry issues norms to guide the health authorities in their planning of health and welfare services, the local authorities are not bound by these. Consequently, the kinds of programs and services provided by the different local authorities are varied. Developing integration and coordination between the local authority health programs and those of the central health department is often difficult. Since there is no statutory provision for coordination, such integration must be developed at the local level by communication and interaction between the Medical Officer of Health and the psychiatric consultants from the hospitals in the area, who then must gain the backing of their respective superiors and governing bodies. Although it is hoped that implementation of the plans for reorganization of the local governments and of the Health Service will ameliorate this problem, it will still be up to each local authority to determine how much it will invest in facilities and programs to provide community care for the mentally ill.

JOINT PROGRAMS

A number of programs of various types have been developed by the mutual participation of hospital and local authority. Such programs are most readily developed in areas where the population served by the hospital coincides with that of the local authority. In such combined efforts, the treatment services (inpatient, outpatient, day-hospital, domiciliary visits, etc.) are provided by the hospital and its consultants, while the "social services" (sheltered workshops, day centers, therapeutic social clubs, half-way hostels, group homes, etc.) are provided by the local health authority. Such arrangements usually involve joint appointment of the psychiatric consultant by the local authority and by the hospital, and frequently some system of joint appointments for social workers as well.

Joint appointments are found in programs largely inaugurated by the local authority, such as in Camden, or in programs largely maintained by the hospital, such as at Mapperley in Nottingham, as well as in general-hospital oriented programs such as in Salford, which illustrates an integrated program initiated by the local authority. The program at Mapperley is an integrated program developed by the hospital. The acme of hospital/local authority integration and coordination is the joint program of the Warlingham Park Hospital and the Croydon Department of Health.

THE GENERAL PRACTITIONER

While both the hospitals and the local authorities have repeatedly proclaimed that the general practitioners are the key figures in any programs of community mental health, neither has done much to translate this idea into reality. For his own part, the general practitioner, with certain notable exceptions, has been reluctant to place himself in the forefront of community mental health efforts (110).

It is the general practitioner's responsibility to make referrals of those patients which he finds are mentally ill. His decision as to when such a referral is necessary will reflect both his attitude toward mental illness and his skill in recognizing it. Those more interested in mental health problems tend to identify and refer patients earlier than do those who seek to avoid problems of mental illness.

Once the general practitioner has identified a patient as mentally ill, several courses of action are open to him. He may refer the patient to a diagnostic outpatient clinic if there is one in the area, or he may notify the mental welfare officer of the patient's problem and ask his help in arranging admission of the patient to a hospital. If he is on good terms with a particular psychiatric consultant, he may call upon him directly to make a domiciliary diagnostic visit to his patient, or may even refer the patient to be seen privately by the consultant. Some general practitioners avoid contact with the psychiatrist entirely, preferring to make referrals to the local-authority social work staff.

When patients are discharged from the mental hospital, the proper procedure is to notify the appropriate general practitioner, who is then expected to follow the patient medically after his return to the community. This aftercare includes regulation of the psychiatric medications prescribed by the hospital, and periodic observation to detect symptoms of returning illness. It is not mandatory, however, for the general practitioner to restore to his list patients who have spent long periods in a mental hospital. Further, the lack of interest shown by many general practitioners for psychiatric problems, coupled with their frequent lack of expertise in the administration of the psychotropic drugs, often leads hospital consultants to prefer to maintain follow-up contact with the patient, either directly through outpatient clinics operated by the hospital, by home visits carried out by the hospital nurses, or, where there is close cooperation with the local authority, by way of their aftercare programs, which generally consist of follow-up by social workers or by the mental welfare officer.

Some general practitioners, and they are a minority, have an interest in psychiatric problems. Courses in psychiatry for general practitioners are conducted by various centers, such as the Tavistock. All but six of the mental hospitals have programs in general-practitioner training.

Four general hospital units operate courses for general practitioners, and 21 others participate in general courses operated by the hospitals as a whole. All university departments of psychiatry take part in the programs for education of general practitioners. There are various types of courses offered to the general practitioner; 36 of them are continuing or occasional courses, 28 are weekend courses, 4 are intensive one-week courses, and 2 are residential courses.

Courses for general practitioners usually are well attended, though some of the instructors are convinced that only a fraction of those participating in the seminars actually employ what they learn in the management of their patients' psychiatric problems. Another fraction are said to attend such courses primarily seeking help with their own personal problems. Some general practitioners, while not taking on additional psychiatric responsibilities as part of their own practice, are nevertheless helped by such courses to identify patients' emotional problems more readily and to be more sophisticated in the process of making psychiatric referrals.

Some local authorities have inaugurated programs setting up "health teams." This involves assigning (seconding) social workers to general practitioners under a variety of arrangements. Most commonly this is done with groups of general practitioners, either those normally practicing together in a group practice or health center or by bringing together several independently practicing general practitioners to form the team. Often midwives, health visitors, and others from the local authority staff participate, in addition to the social worker. Health teams may meet at regular or irregular intervals to discuss the problems of the general practitioner's patients, for whom assistance from the local authority staff is sought. At times the local authority social workers or others use these meetings to obtain medical advice from the general practitioner with regard to their clients' problems. One such arrangement is found in Salford.

Because the community programs in Britain have developed largely in conjunction with efforts to promote discharge of long-stay hospital patients, these programs have emphasized rehabilitation and resocialization far more than those in many American communities. The general-hospital-based programs, as well as some others, have also emphasized rapid treatment and high patient turnover. In any event the consequence of these efforts has been a sharp reduction in the number of new long-stay patients.

Evaluative studies relevant to community mental health are being conducted primarily at the Social Psychiatry Research Unit of the Medical Research Council, under Dr. John Wing, located at the Maudsley Institute for Psychiatry; and the Clinical Psychiatry Research Unit based at Graylingwell Hospital, Chichester, under Dr. Peter Sainsbury.

6

Specialized service segments

As has been noted, the number of mental hospital beds, for long-stay patients particularly, is expected to undergo a considerable decrease by 1975 (91). This is to be accompanied by a significant increase in the number of general-hospital psychiatric beds, chiefly for short-stay and medium-stay patients, in addition to an anticipated development of additional community facilities.

The reduction of psychiatric beds in the institutions is dependent upon two factors: first, a sharp decrease in the generation of new long-stay cases; second, the clearing-out of the mental hsopitals by mobilization and discharge to the community of the chronically ill patient who has been in the hospital for many years. A number of specialized services have been developed over a period of years, the utilization of which contributes to the realization of these goals.

MENTAL HOSPITAL OPERATED SERVICES

Inpatient Service

"The Open Door"

Some years ago, in the post-World-War-II period, it occurred to several administrators of the mental hospitals that it might be possible to unlock the doors, giving patients, at the very least, freedom of the hospital grounds. It is not certain who originated this idea, but Dr. T. P. Rees at the Warlingham Park Hospital in Croydon was certainly responsible for publicizing it on a grand scale, thus calling it to the attention of many other hospital superintendents who were thereby stimulated to employ similar approaches. In most instances, patients were given the freedom to leave the grounds of the hospital and venture into the nearby towns.

The utilization of the "open door policy" brought the mental patient into contact with the communities. Those who were permitted such freedom prior to the use of tranquilizing drugs tended to be the more withdrawn and apathetic chronically ill patients who were, in any event, neither dangerous nor a menace to the community. These experiments served to condition the community to the presence of the chronic mentally ill and to reduce their fear and suspicion of such patients. In fact, communities participating in the pioneering experiments, such as that of Warlingham Park, derived a significant sense of gratification and feeling of accomplishment. It may well be that Croydon's early experience as a pioneering community in the implementation of the open door policy had a significant positive effect upon its subsequent development of progressive programs for the community treatment of the mentally ill.

The Therapeutic Community

Likewise in the framework of the circumstances following World War II, the therapeutic-community idea was developed by Maxwell Jones at the Henderson Hospital in Sutton, Surrey (71). This program was originally established in 1947 as part of an effort in the treatment of psychopaths, as the "social rehabilitation unit" of the Belmont Hospital. The unit became autonomous in 1959, and was renamed Henderson Hospital. The focus here is on increased responsibility on the part of the patients in determining their own therapeutic program, the assumption being that such a move would tend to counter irresponsibility or anti-social behavior. There was a considerable utilization of group psychotherapy, and because of limitations of nursing staff, social workers were utilized extensively in the therapeutic program.

These innovations stressed resocialization and rehabilitation, demonstrated that patients could assume larger amounts of independent responsibility (and incidentally suggested that it might be possible to operate an active program with fewer staff by so doing), and introduced greater flexibility into the therapeutic team roles.

The therapeutic-community approach has received wide publicity and has been incorporated, with variations, into many programs. These range from programs almost completely determined by patient decisions ("patient self-government") to those based on an active participation by staff and patients in daily features of ward living ("milieu therapy"). Many utilize extensive group (patient and staff) discussion ("therapeutic community conferences") in the treatment of patients of every diagnostic category and description.

Rehabilitation Wards

With the growing emphasis in hospitals upon mobilizing institutionalized, long-stay chronically ill patients in preparation for discharge into the community, institutions began to re-evaluate their chronic patients, collect those potentially suitable for rehabilitation from the various back wards, and bring them together in a common unit, generally termed a "rehabilitation ward." Transfer to such a ward thus came to connote the last step of hospitalization prior to return to the community. Rehabilitation wards tended to be staffed better than most "back wards" of the hospital and reflected enthusiasm and high morale. Considerable effort was invested in resocialization and rehabilitation activities, particularly in the industrial sense.

Preparation for discharge did not necessarily mean preparation for return to full independent life within the community. Some patients might return to be community wards of their families, who would take over from the hospital the burden of looking after the chronically ill patient. Others might be expected to live in sheltered accommodations, such as half-way hostels. Some patients might go directly from the hospital to some form of employment either in open industry or in a sheltered workshop. Others might require continuing therapeutic contact such as day hospitals or day social centers.

Generally speaking, there is no anticipated time limit for the patient's stay on the rehabilitation ward. Some patients might respond to the "total push" effort rapidly and be ready to resume some sort of constructive community employment within a short time; other patients respond much more slowly, some remaining on rehabilitation wards for several years. Generally, the medical and nursing staff tend not to "give up" on patients who have been moved to rehabilitation wards but continue to work with them in the hope of finally moving them out of the hospital. Only rarely are patients moved back from rehabilitation wards to the back wards whence they came.

Industrial Therapy

One of the programs most widely used in conjunction with the rehabilitation wards and the efforts at returning patients to the community has been industrial therapy. Industrial rehabilitation activities have been centered within the community as well as in the hospital itself. Industrial therapy developed out of the occupational therapy programs of the hospitals with, however, the special objective of preparing the patients for the experience of holding down some form of industrial employment, thereby facilitating their chances for a successful return to the community. Industrial therapy programs, therefore, attempt to simulate the conditions to be found in factories. Patients, even while still in the hospital, are expected to turn up for "work" on time and on their own initiative; to have a regard for the quality of the work that they produce; and to progress from simpler to more complex and difficult tasks. Regular assessments made of the patient's work performance, and credited to him, reflect the progress he is making and encourage him to further effort. They also serve as indicators of the patient's readiness for discharge and his potential for holding down a job.

Yet another, and perhaps a major, incentive for the patient's participation and interest is that of pay. The work done in the industrial therapy workshops is contracted for with local industry by a member of the staff serving as industrial manager. The company pays the hospital for work successfully completed, usually at lower than commercial rates. This provides sufficient funds, however, for the patients to be remunerated according to the volume and quality of the work turned out. In some instances elaborate scales of pay have been worked out. The pay scale generally ranges from several new pence to £2.00 per week.

While it is not necessary for a large remuneration to be paid to the hospital for the work done by patients in the industrial therapy program, it is important that they are not exploited. Consequently, the industrial manager tries to obtain a good "price" for the patient-produced items that will be not too far below the commercial rate. On the other hand, he is faced with the problem of maintaining a continuity of task assignments. This requires having a number of contracts available, so that there are no periods of idleness when a particular job has been completed. This occasionally makes it necessary to accept certain kinds of contracts at lower rates. These are often for producing items used by the hospital, by a group of hospitals, or by other charitable organizations. Graylingwell Hospital, for example, turns out all of the sterilized packs of bandages and other sterile goods used by the entire Chichester group of hospitals.

The background of the industrial manager is sometimes that of an occupational therapist, but may vary considerably. Often he has had some experience in industry. The types of contracts negotiated for by the industrial manager will frequently reflect his own skills and background. Contractual work may be merely folding and packing previously manufactured items, light assembling tasks, or more complex operations requiring the use of specialized machinery which is generally supplied by the company.

Since it has been an almost universal experience of the contracting companies that the quality of work is at least as good as that in the average factory, most well-operated industrial therapy workshops now have little difficulty in securing contracts, although seasonal factors sometimes limit the amount of work available.

The Disablement Resettlement Officer (DRO). An important aspect of the industrial rehabilitation program is finding the patient a job when he is ready to return to the community. Some patients may even begin employment in outside industry while still residing in the mental hospital. Such employment is generally arranged for by the Disablement Resettlement Officer, an employee of the Department of Employment and Productivity (formerly the Ministry of Labour). The Disablement Resettlement Officer (DRO) visits the hospital industrial workshops, meets with the patients and the industrial therapy manager, and familiarizes himself with the skills and potentials of the patients awaiting return to the community. He keeps himself informed about opportunities for employment in industry, so that he can expedite job placement when a patient is ready and there is a suitable opening.

When the industrial therapy programs were first initiated, job placements of the first groups of patients to be discharged were quite successful; these were the long-stay patients with the greatest potential for rehabilitation. Many were able to accept community employment, and only a few had to leave their jobs or return to the hospital. Later groups of patients have not been so successful. Returns to the hospitals have been higher, but the overall program continues to function on an acceptable level. During 1970, of 178,370 mental hospital admissions in England, 113,226 were readmissions of previously discharged patients (38). Most often failures at job placements are due not to lack of job skills but rather to difficulties in the social sphere, such as getting on with other workers, relating to authority, or maintaining acceptable attendance records.

The degree to which hospitals have developed industrial therapy programs varies widely. In some hospitals work programs are still a minor part of the rehabilitation efforts; in others, such as Cheadle Royal, the industrial therapy program has become, in fact, a hospital-based factory which markets its own products instead of contracting with industry for projects.

Industrial Therapy Units. A good example of an industrial-therapy unit is to be found at Graylingwell Hospital, in Chichester, where the unit is run on the lines of a factory, and patients clock in and out on their own responsibility. Work assessments are made on each patient, and the patients are classified into grades according to their capacities. Patients are paid by the hour, the rate varying with the grade. Reassessments are made weekly during the first six weeks and then repeated whenever the staff considers it necessary. Regular staff meetings are held to check on the patients' progress.

Dr. Capstick, the psychiatric consultant in charge, believes that assessment not only helps the staff to recognize improvements in the patient, it also turns the patient's own attention to the progress he is making and serves to motivate him to improve. The remuneration rate, which is linked to his grade and therefore reflects the gains he has made, is used by the patient as an indicator of his own readiness to leave the hospital.

Approximately 200 patients work in the industrial therapy unit, of whom 80 come from the rehabilitation wards of the hospital and most of the remainder from various other parts of the institution. They normally work 5 hours a day, though more active patients may put in 7 hours.

Work flows steadily through the unit, with about 10 different kinds of work-tasks done simultaneously by different patient groups. Most jobs call for hand work, but some require special equipment supplied by the contracting firms. A group of 30-40 patients inspects and packs the plastic bottles made by other patients, discarding the rejects. Other patients make and sell seed-boxes and grow and sell fruits and vegetables in their own garden. They also make and sell decorative concrete tiles for garden walls.

The quality of workmanship is quite high. The patients do some work for export; they even inspect plastic work done in regular factories. Those doing inspection or serving as checkers are in the highest grade, and patients are very eager to achieve this status.

At Mapperley Hospital in Nottingham the industrial therapy program serves approximately 50 inpatients and over 100 day patients. The day hospital emphasis is reflected in its name, which is the Day Unit for Industrial Therapy (DUIT). There are 10 staff people on the unit, which is run like a factory; patients clock in and out on their own responsibility and are paid on a piece-work basis.

There is a regular flow of contract work on the unit; some work is occasionally turned down. Activities include packing ladies' underwear, carding pencils, packaging eyebrow pencils, assembling pens, wrapping "wickets" in polyethylene bags, etc. They do furniture repairs for the hospital, and stain and polish furniture made by the Institute for the Blind. They operate a complete print shop, where all the hospital's printing is done, and a shoe repair shop. Even the day hospital dining room is operated as a canteen run by the patients.

The DRO visits the unit each week to study the patients' work abilities and tries to find jobs for patients considered ready for outside employment. Seventy-five patients were placed in industrial jobs during the first year of operation of the unit; very few returned to the hospital. Subsequent patient groups have not done as well, however, and now around 40% of those placed are unable to hold their job. The hospital staff are hopeful that the community will build a sheltered workshop for those patients unable to adjust to regular industrial work.

Social Therapy

In some hospitals, programs stressing resocialization have been developed in addition to the industrial therapy programs. Such units, called "social therapy" or "psychotherapy" units, emphasize group activities involving social interaction between patients and staff. Group psychotherapy is often utilized in conjunction with these programs. The Graylingwell social therapy unit and the Mapperley and Littlemore psychotherapy units illustrate this type of program.

Partial Hospitalization

In some instances patients discharged from 24-hour hospitalization continue to require considerable supervision or treatment. At some hospitals, patients living in the community, either with their own families or in sheltered accommodations such as hostels or group homes, may return to the mental hospital during the daytime hours.

The idea of partial hospitalization was introduced to England by Dr. Joshua Bierer in the late 1940's (5). The first day-hospital in Britain was the Marlborough Day Hospital, which he founded and which was taken over as a unit of the National Health Service in 1948. The effectiveness of partial hospitalization in reducing the number of beds required for 24-hour hospitalization has, over the years, been well demonstrated, and the idea has been widely adopted with variations.

Many mental hospitals operate so-called day-hospital units. These may be separate self-contained facilities providing exclusively for patients residing in the community, such as the Maudsley Day Hospital. Other hospitals utilize their regular inpatient facilities for day-time programs for discharged patients living in the community. At Graylingwell, for example, the day patients are assigned to programs identical to those of the regular inpatients, and within any group of activities, one cannot distinguish between those patients resident at the hospital and those living in the community. Similarly at Littlemore Hospital, particularly in the Phoenix Unit, the admixture of day patients and inpatients becomes homogenized; in fact at the time of my visit to Littlemore, all but one of the patients participating in the Phoenix Unit program were day patients. Other hospitals provide distinct programs for day patients and inpatients, but conduct them more or less within the same general facilities as for example, at Mapperley Hospital at Nottingham.

A day hospital within the community of East Croydon is housed in facilities jointly operated by the local authority and the Warlingham Park Hospital. It is entirely off hospital grounds and easily accessible to community residents. It is utilized for patients who have never been hospitalized, as well as for those discharged from the hospital.

The Marlborough Day Hospital, affiliated neither with a mental hospital nor with any local authority, is a completely autonomous unit operated under the Health Service. Since it serves no particular catchment area, its patients may come from considerable distances. In recent years, a number of inpatient beds have been added to the day-hospital facilities, so that full-time hospitalization can now also be provided for a small number of patients. The Marlborough Day Hospital is unique, too, in that it provides certain services for children, which are not usually provided at other such facilities.

Because of the distance of the hospital from the community or for other reasons, a patient may be unable to make his daily return to the hospital on his own. He may then be brought to the hospital by ambulance provided by the local authority. This service is intended primarily for aged patients attending day-care programs, but it may be given to other kinds of patients. All patients participating in the day-hospital program at the Queen's Park Hospital Psychiatric Unit in Blackburn are bussed back and forth each day by the local authority ambulances.

The hospital may also be used as a hostel or "night hospital" for patients working in the community during the day, especially where the local authorities have failed to provide adequate sheltered living accommodations for discharged mental patients.

"Psychogeriatrics"

The use of the institution as a day hospital has particular value in the treatment of so-called "psychogeriatric" cases. Aged patients are often regarded by the administrators of the mental institutions as major impediments to their rehabilitation programs. An increasing number of senile and arteriosclerotic patients, incapable of rehabilitation, tend to live longer than in the past and accumulate in the hospitals. Although most administrators advocate care in special geriatric hospitals for these patients, some are ready to accept responsibility for those aged patients having clear-cut psychiatric syndromes. Others feel that even these patients should be treated in "psychogeriatric units" of specialized geriatric hospitals which would be visited by psychiatric consultants in an advisory capacity. The Mapperley Hospital in Nottingham has developed a rather comprehensive program which uses the institution as a day hospital for the elderly, including the senile and those with specific psychiatric syndromes. A full gamut of services is provided.

Recently the Society of Clinical Psychiatrists reviewed the care of the aged mentally ill and made a number of recommendations (23).

Domiciliary Visits

Although it is quite uncommon in the United States for the psychiatrist to visit the mental patient in his home, this service has become a standard procedure in Britain. Such domiciliary visits are always made by the psychiatric consultant and never by junior psychiatric staff. For the most part, the staff are limited to a single diagnostic visit. Consultants receive added remuneration for such visits beyond their regular compensation. If the consultant is full time with the hospital service, he is not paid for the first eight domiciliary visits made in any one quarter. Most hospital consultants are on "maximum part time" with the Health Service (9/11 time), spend the remainder of their time in private practice, and are therefore eligible to receive payment for every domiciliary visit. There is, however, a maximum of £1,100 that may be paid for domiciliary visits during one year.

Diagnostic domiciliary visits may be arranged with the consultant either directly by the general practitioner or the mental welfare officer referring the patient. If, following such a domiciliary consultation, it is decided that the patient requires hospitalization, he is assigned in the hospital to the care of the consultant who made the initial evaluation.

"The Worthing Experiment"

While most domiciliary visits are limited to a single home call, the program initiated by Dr. Joshua Carse of the Graylingwell Hospital included repeated therapeutic visits to the homes of mentally ill people (10, 11, 12). This was the so-called "Worthing Experiment," conducted in the community of Worthing, about 20 miles from Chichester, one of the areas for which the Graylingwell Hospital has responsibility. The aim of Dr. Carse's experiment, carried out prior to the advent of tranquilizers, was to treat as many patients as possible within their own homes, without admission to the hospital. The psychiatrist made repeated visits to the home, gave guidance and advice about care to the patient's relatives, and attempted some therapeutic intervention and supportive work with the patient himself. On this basis Carse was able to avoid admitting some patients who otherwise would have been hospitalized, many of them as long-stay patients. Carse's experiment did not involve the local authority services, nor was there particular preparation of the community for this project; consequently considerable resentment and resistance developed in certain quarters to the experiment. Nevertheless, this program which was continued only for a specified period of time (hence "experiment"), demonstrated the feasibility of maintaining patients out of the hospital. In its final year, it reduced admissions to Graylingwell by 59% without obvious serious consequences (62).

Domiciliary Visits by Nurses

In some hospitals, aftercare and follow-up of discharged patients are provided through domiciliary visits by hospital nurses (3, 81, 82, 111). Such programs are generally most suitable for hospitals fairly near the communities they serve and are perhaps best suited to general hospitals. In addition to the distance the nurse must travel to see her assigned patients, there is the question of adequate numbers of staff. A theoretical premise which helped to develop the practice of domiciliary visits by nurses was that patients in the hospital tend to establish useful therapeutic relationships with the nurses responsible for their care, and it is desirable to maintain this relationship following discharge. In practice, however, the nurse making domiciliary visits usually does not visit the patient for whom she was responsible in the hospital. In many instances nurses on domiciliary service do not have simultaneous in-hospital responsibilities. Domiciliary visiting is usually either a regular full-time assignment or is done on a rotation basis (nurses taking it for a specific number of months, then returning to hospital duties, turning over the domiciliary caseload to another nurse).

The use of nurses for domiciliary visits has sometimes aroused friction with social workers, who customarily have regarded aftercare home visits as falling within their professional province. An argument favoring the use of nurses is that they are able to provide necessary treatment similar to what they might render in the hospital, including medication. With the increasingly widespread use of long-acting Fluphenazine preparations (Modecate*), injections of tranquilizers are commonly administered by nurses making domiciliary visits.

Occasionally friction has developed between the hospital-based psychiatric nurse and the public health nurse over the responsibility for making domiciliary home visits to former patients of the mental hospital. Here the argument favoring the use of the psychiatric nurse rests upon her ability to recognize psychiatric syndromes and particularly upon her ability to evaluate the possible necessity of returning the patient to inpatient status.

*Modecate is the trade name in Great Britain for Fluphenazine decanoate marked by E. R. Squibb & Sons.

Some people consider that the use of psychiatric nurses to make domiciliary visits wastes time. They prefer the arrangement where discharged patients residing in the community come to the hospital for follow-up, where they are then seen by the psychiatric nurse as outpatients. The nurse performs at the hospital those duties she would otherwise perform during a domiciliary visit. Interestingly, there have been objections to the performance of these duties by the nurse in the hospital setting, whereas there has been general approbation for their performance of the same functions in the patient's home—this despite the fact that the nurse is much more readily supervised in the hospital setting and has available to her the other resources of the hospital and staff members whose assistance she may call upon. Those who favor the domiciliary visit point out that the nurse can evaluate the total living arrangement, family interaction, etc., when visiting the patient's home, which she could not do if she saw the patient at the hospital. In many instances these patients are living in marginal circumstances in sheltered accommodations, and the home visit helps the nurse to determine if the patient is being adequately cared for and nourished and if his basic needs have been attended to.

An extensive program of domiciliary visits is conducted in Croydon by nurses from Warlingham Park Hospital. In some cases, the nurse does not make regular domiciliary visits but will make home calls as follow-up in the event a patient has failed to appear for a regular attendance at a day hospital.

DISTRICT GENERAL HOSPITAL SERVICES

The experience of the Manchester Regional Hospital Board has been used to support the claim that a marked reduction in the number of mental hospital beds can be expected by 1975 (28). The Manchester ratio of psychiatric beds to population has been consistently lower than the national average ever since the inauguration of the program utilizing psychiatric units in general hospitals. Programs in the Manchester region, such as the one at Queen's Park Hospital in Blackburn, have demonstrated further that general hospital-based psychiatric services can provide the full treatment needs of all psychiatric patients from the designated catchment area, with the possible exception of the senile, and "psychogeriatric" population (102, 103). Even where the general hospital does not seek to carry the entire load, the number of institutional beds required is sharply reduced (7, 9, 18, 65). Nevertheless, it seems to be the ambition of most general hospitals to provide all mental health services for an entire catchment area using a much smaller number of beds than would be the case were the area being served by the mental institution (2).

The general hospital is a most rational focus for community psychiatry programs. Its location in the midst of the urban community makes it more readily accessible than the remote mental institutions. This means not only that hospital-based day-treatment programs, industrial therapy workshops, and clinics are easily accessible to discharged inpatients requiring continuing care, but that help is available earlier in the course of an illness and that new cases can be recognized more promptly. By means of early case finding and timely therapeutic intervention, regressive defensive patterns leading to chronic clinical pictures can be aborted. Thus, the general hospital psychiatric program can contribute to the preventive as well as the rehabilitative aspects of community mental health efforts (14, 91).

Generally speaking, the psychiatric services in the general hospitals are not integrated with the other medical and surgical services of the hospital. Very often the psychiatric facilities are in a separate building and are "part" of the general hospital by virtue of being on the same grounds rather than because of any interaction or integration of their activities with those of the hospital proper.

The proximity of general hospital services, however, does facilitate the ready transfer of those psychiatric patients requiring treatment for physical illness during the course of their hospitalization, and likewise makes available to the general hospital the services of the psychiatric consultant as well as facilities for prompt transfer of those patients who develop psychiatric complications in the course of their somatic illnesses.

Most of the psychiatric units in general hospitals have been developed in facilities converted from other functions; many are in the old poor-law sections of the general hospitals. A few general hospital psychiatric units, such as the one at St. Mary Abbots Hospital in London, have been built for that purpose. The size of the unit varies considerably from only a few beds to over 100. Indeed some of the larger units seem to be almost autonomous psychiatric hospitals on the grounds of a general hospital.

The units also vary significantly in their patterns of function. They tend to have fewer staff than their medical or surgical counterparts in the general hospital (2). In some instances the facilities must be shared with other services (as at Salford where the ward is shared with geriatric patients). The Blackburn facilities are organized in traditional mental-hospital fashion, with separate male and female sections each with admitting wards and wards for short-, medium-, and long-stay patients. Electroshock therapy and drugs are used and vigorous greatment and early discharge are emphasized.

Recently a directive from the Health Ministry recommended a complete transfer of psychiatric inpatient treatment from mental institutions to general hospital psychiatric units and gradual phasing-out of the mental hospitals (42).

Despite its focus on the general hospital, the emphasis is still on rehabilitation rather than prevention, although the Health Ministry stresses the importance of providing the full range of treatment with as little interference as possible to the patient's ordinary way of life. In a service of this kind, most of the patient's treatment may take place while he lives in the community. The memorandum consists of three main elements: one is the provision in the district general hospital or group of general hospitals providing a district service, of a department for the mentally ill (including day patient and outpatient services) serving a defined local geographical district, preferably that corresponding to the district served by the other departments of the hospital or group of hospitals. This has advantages of ready cooperation between the psychiatric department and other departments and easy access to the full range of diagnostic and other facilities of a general hospital. Another main element is the provision of adequate community services by local authorities, social work services, homes for the elderly, hostels, and group homes, or other supervised lodgings. The third main element is the joint planning, development, and operation of services. This calls for, among other things, the setting up of "therapeutic teams" which will include a consultant psychiatrist, medical staff, nurses, occupational therapists, and social workers. Some members of the team will often be on the staff of the local authority. Where social workers are employed by the hospital, it is expected that they will work closely with local-authority social services staff and that psychologists and clinical psychotherapists will also be available. For the plan to succeed, the team will have to develop a close relationship with the family doctors, district nurses, health visitors, and volunteer workers, as well as officers of the local probation, disablement resettlement, and social security services. Each team will be responsible for a defined geographical area of about 60,000 population within the district served by the hospital group and will be based on a 30-bed ward (42).

The plan calls for the initial steps in organizing the transition to be taken within the framework of existing services. The catchment area of each hospital for the mentally ill may be split into the geographical districts served by the general hospital groups in that catchment area. As new admissions to the mental hospital cease, the patients remaining in the mental hospital will increasingly consist of elderly long-stay patients, emphasizing the need for close links with geriatric hospitals, with geriatric general hospital departments, and with local authority services for the elderly.

Because it provides active treatment for all patients, and a higher proportion are treated as day patients or outpatients, a general hospital psychiatry department requires higher staff/inpatient ratios, especially for nurses, than the mental hospital. As far as possible, the new departments are expected to be staffed by transferring personnel from the mental hospitals. Maintaining morale of staff who remain at the mental hospital will be a prime responsibility of hospital authorities. It is believed that a well-planned and coordinated program of transition, fully explained to all staff at the outset, can avoid unwarranted fears about future employment. Management will need to foster a multi-disciplinary approach and to keep the medical and nurse staffing organization under regular review. All undergraduate teaching hospitals are also expected to provide comprehensive services for the full range of mentally ill patients for a defined district.

The memorandum expresses the belief that a suitably designed ward in the general hospital can accommodate all or most adult mentally ill patients in a system of progressive patient care (42). Day hospitals, able to provide care for all types of patients, can be developed in a general hospital even before psychiatric beds become available. Ambulant inpatients can also share the use of the day hospital for occupational, social, and recreational facilities (see Outpatient Services).

Personal contact and cooperation between hospital and local authority staff is considered essential. Hospital staffs are advised to maintain close contact with Directors of Social Services and their staff, in view of their community health responsibilities and general advisory role, and with Medical Officers of Health and their staff. The Local Authority Social Services Department is responsible for finding suitable residential accommodations, such as hostels, group homes, supervised lodgings, and social work support for patients discharged from the hospital. Local-authority social workers are usually in the best position to arrange admission to local-authority accommodations and to find and supervise suitable landladies. Social work services will continue to be needed to provide support for the patient and his family. The therapeutic relationship with the psychiatric nurse also is considered to be vital to the recovery and continuing good health of many patients.

The department of psychiatry in the general hospital is expected to provide consultation, assessment, and treatment for drug- or alcohol-dependent patients referred to it, although special units, such as alcohol- or drug-withdrawal clinics may be necessary.

Outpatient Services

Outpatient services may be operated either by a mental hospital or a psychiatric unit of a general hospital. Often, the clinics are held at community general hospitals but conducted by consultants from the mental hospitals. The major emphasis is usually on diagnosis. Patients referred by general practitioners, social agencies, and mental welfare officers receive psychiatric examination and psychological tests. Following such evaluation a patient may either be admitted to a hospital or assigned to one of the alternative treatment programs.

In addition to the diagnostic services, most outpatient services offer a variety of treatment activities. Ambulatory electroshock therapy is frequently used. It is administered generally twice a week; the patients come in the morning, receive their treatment, are given an opportunity to recover from the acute effects, and are then returned home.

Outpatient clinics also frequently provide treatment with psychotropic drugs. Either they are administered at the clinic by injection, given by the nurse, as in the case of the long-acting Fluphenazine preparations, or the patients come in periodically for adjustment and regulation of oral medication prescribed by the doctor. A number of studies show that approximately one-half of the ambulatory patients do not take their oral psychotropic medications regularly; hence there has been an increasing tendency to utilize the long-acting preparations which are administered parenterally (42).

Some outpatient clinics also provide group psychotherapy, particularly in settings where there is an active training program. Such psychotherapy is generally conducted by the registrar and occasionally by other members of the mental health team. It is less often conducted by the psychiatric consultant. Individual psychotherapy is minimal; when given it is usually supportive, with patients who come at intervals varying from once a week to once in several months. The therapeutic session generally ranges between 15 minutes and a half-hour. Much psychotherapy is done in the name of "casework" by social workers. Intensive individual psychotherapy is extremely rare.

24-Hour Emergency Services

Ordinarily psychiatric emergencies are seen by the general practitioner. If he is unable to deal with the situation on his own, he has available to him the services of the mental welfare officer who is usually on call 24 hours per day, 7 days a week. The mental welfare officer in turn has access to the services of the psychiatric consultant, who is available to make a domiciliary visit. Consequently there is a significantly smaller tendency to have 24-hour emergency psychiatric services at hospitals in Britain than in the United States. Where such services are available, as at the Maudsley or at Salford, patients and referring agencies increasingly attempt to circumvent the general practitioner by applying for psychiatric services directly through the psychiatric emergency facility.

A 24-hour emergency service is maintained by the psychiatric unit at St. Mary Abbots, a general hospital in central London serving a catchment area in the borough of Kensington-Chelsea with a population of

130,000. This service is used by police of the area to "dump" all sorts of problems, including drunks and addicts. The unit also receives a large number of transients who have no local general practitioner. The transients are mainly young foreign nationals who have arrived via the West London Air Terminal located in the area and who present a variety of psychiatric syndromes.

The Health Ministry's memorandum has stated that emergency psychiatric consultation services should be available at all district general hospitals (42).

LOCAL AUTHORITY COMMUNITY SERVICES

Local authorities are required under statutory obligation to provide for prevention of illness, for care and aftercare of the sick, and for aid to the handicapped.

These services vary widely in quality and quantity. In the realm of mental health they may include, in addition to the statutory services for the mentally retarded and the mental welfare officer's statutory duties of expediting mental hospital admissions and post-discharge follow-up and aftercare, the provision of sheltered workshops, occupational centers, social centers, therapeutic social clubs, and sheltered living accommodations such as group homes or hostels for the mentally ill. In addition, the social work staff often provides casework and psychotherapy. A psychiatric consultant from a nearby mental or general hospital, who holds a part-time joint appointment with the local authority, nominally supervises these activities. Most local authority services for the mentally ill are rehabilitative, rather than preventive.

For the most part, services for children are separate from the regular mental health provisions. In a few local authorities, child guidance clinics have been encompassed within the mental health section of the Health Department, but this is the exception rather than the rule.

Although the Health Ministry issues norms to guide the local authorities in planning health and welfare services, the local authorities are not bound by them; hence the variation in programs and services. Integrating and coordinating local-authority health programs with those of the central health department may also be difficult. Since there is no statutory provision for coordination, such integration at the local level must be developed by communication and interaction between the Medical Officer of Health and the psychiatric consultants from the hospitals in the area, who then must gain the backing of their respective superiors and governing bodies.

The problem has been intensified since the creation of the new

Social Service Department. Now the local-authority mental health services are no longer under medical auspices but are strictly a social service responsibility. In order to effect continuity of care, it is now necessary for the medically oriented hospital staff to relate to and gain the cooperation and collaboration of a separate organization, jealous of its professional prerogatives. With the implementation of the health service reorgnization on April 1, 1974, even the hospital social workers will be transferred to the Social Service Department, further complicating the problems of continuity of care.

Sheltered Workshops

The local authority has statutory responsibility to provide community-based industrial rehabilitation services. Such facilities as have been developed by various local authorities are mostly utilized for programs dealing with the mentally retarded rather than the mentally ill. Several local authorities, however, do provide sheltered workshops or industrial rehabilitation services for psychiatric patients. In Camden Borough an industrial therapy unit is operated in a day center under local authority auspices; a similar program is conducted in the Borough of Croydon.

The industrial therapy unit is similar to its hospital counterpart in that it is geared towards employment in industry. There is an ongoing work assessment program in which the participants are paid for their work in accordance with their productivity. The pay ranges from 25 new pence to £2.00 per week, the latter being the maximum allowed under the social security benefits programs. The aim is to move the patients into jobs as quickly as possible.

The sheltered workshops, on the other hand, are geared for rehabilitation through work, providing a sheltered facility where the community-based patient performs industrial work as a form of occupational therapy. He may receive remuneration for work done, but the demands are not as stringent as those in the industrial therapy units. Sheltered workshops usually allow patients to attend for long periods of time, since these patients are usually unable to sustain themselves independently in an industrial situation. Frequently they are patients who have tried to hold jobs in the community but have been unsuccessful for a variety of reasons. At times these patients are quite skilled and the quality of work performed may be quite high, but they are unable to keep jobs because of their inability to maintain a social adjustment in the work situation.

The Department of Employment and Productivity likewise maintains a number of industrial rehabilitation units, established essentially to assist the physically handicapped. It was the early experience of these units that 25% of the patients working in them had psychiatric problems as their primary disability. Since the Ministry considered that the presence of psychiatric patients tended to slow the units down, they have subsequently restricted the utilization of these facilities by psychiatric patients.

Hostels

Hostels are sheltered living accommodations in the community. The local authority has the statutory responsibility to provide this type of accommodation. Hostels may be provided for the mentally subnormal or the mentally ill. Some hostels admit both types of residents.

The half-way hostel for the mentally ill patient discharged from hospital may be operated directly by the local authority, or the local authority may purchase the services of a hostel operated by some voluntary agency, such as the Richmond Fellowship or the Mental After-Care Association (MACA).

The hostels are generally converted houses with group living accommodations for 10 to 30 residents. While there are occasional single rooms, most of the residents sleep in dormitories accommodating 2 or 3 people. Both men and women live in the same hostel. The residents of a given hostel are usually selected on the basis of common personality characteristics and problems, age, chronicity, etc. The person in charge of the hostel, called the warden, generally lives at the hostel. He is assisted by the bursar. The residents participate in maintaining the hostel, perform the household chores, and often do the marketing and cooking as well. There is generally a fixed food budget, within which the menus are decided upon by the residents. In hostels where most of the residents work during the day, there may be a paid cook.

Patients unable to support themselves receive a social security grant which includes an amount to cover the expenses of living accommodations. These funds are paid to the hostels as the patients' rent and board fee. Those residents of hostels who are able to work and earn sufficient monies, pay their own way out of their earnings.

The hostel at Salford is an illustration of a hostel operated by a local authority. The Kensington Hostel of the Richmond Fellowship is an illustration of a hostel operated by a voluntary organization. The Richmond Fellowship and the MACA are the major voluntary groups operating hostels for former mental patients.

Group Homes

A group home is another form of sheltered living accommodation, with less structure than the hostel. Here groups of patients live on their own responsibility. There is no warden, bursar, or cook. The residents assume all of the household duties and tasks, deciding among themselves how these tasks are to be distributed and performed. Group homes may be owned by the local authority, or they may be premises rented from a landlady who has agreed to provide such accommodations for former hospital patients. Patients discharged to group homes are rather carefully selected because of the responsibility involved. Salford and Croydon local authorities own group homes for former psychiatric inpatients. Graylingwell Hospital sends selected discharged patients to landlady-operated group homes in Chichester, with which it has made special arrangements. Payments for living accommodations in the group homes are made by the local authority through the social-security scheme, as in the case of the hostels.

Aftercare

The local authority also has statutory responsibility for providing aftercare for the mentally ill. The actual provision of such services varies, however. In some areas the general practitioner is expected to assume this function. In other areas aftercare is provided by the mental hospital, the psychiatric service in the general hospital, or through outpatient clinics. Where the local authority provides aftercare, the service may take the form of casework conducted by the staff of the Social Service Department, or follow-up visits to the former patients in their homes by social workers or mental welfare officers. Aftercare may also be carried out at day centers or via social clubs.

Day Centers

While "day hospitals" usually provide the full gamut of treatment facilities available at the mental hospital, including administration of drugs and electroshock therapy, and are therefore under medical auspices, a number of community facilities providing day programs without medical treatment have been developed under the auspices of the local authority. "Day centers" have been established for certain catchment areas, including Camden Borough, Newham, and Salford. Such centers may provide the typical occupational therapy activities or even a full-scale industrial rehabilitation workshop. Other day-center programs include resocialization activities, group therapy, recreational facilities, trips to places of interest, and sponsorship of therapeutic social clubs. Centers may be run by industrial therapists, industrial managers, or occupational therapists; they are often operated by individuals with personal resources but no specific formal training. The staffing pattern will vary according to the particular setting and its goals. Overall supervision generally is provided by the social work staff of the Local Authority Social Service Department.

Social Clubs

Therapeutic social clubs are formed by groups of former hospital patients who meet at regular intervals (generally about once a week) for group discussion and social purposes. The club is often named for the particular day of the week on which it meets, for example, the Wednesday Club or the Sunday Club, etc. The membership of such clubs tends to be quite large, although only a certain fraction attends meetings with any degree of regularity. Others, however, tend to drop in now and then when they feel like it. The clubs provide a degree of social contact which would be otherwise unavailable to these socially isolated former patients. Some club members have retained their membership over the years.

Social clubs may be sponsored by voluntary organizations (e.g., the Camden Mental Health Association), local authority centers (Camden, Newham, etc.), or in conjunction with day hospitals (Marlborough Day), or mental hospitals. Regardless of sponsorship, the focus of the social club is never medical, although meetings are generally attended by social workers and occasionally by psychiatrists or other members of the mental health team.

Meetings are conducted by club officers elected by the members. The activities of the club are planned and carried out by committees which may or may not be assisted by professional staff or volunteers. Activities vary. Some clubs participate in occupational therapy activities available at a particular center; others take trips to places of interest; still others emphasize group discussion. Generally some food, usually tea and sandwiches or cakes, is served at club meetings.

Ambulance Services

Provision of ambulance services is the responsibility of local authorities. In some instances this marks the sole extent of participation by the local authority in the community mental health program. Ambulances are used not only to transport acutely ill patients to the hospital but also to bus people to and from day hospitals or day centers. Their major use in this field has been for the psychogeriatric patient but in some areas, such as Blackburn, they may be used also to transport other psychiatric patients to the day hospital.

Home Helps

If a woman becomes ill and is not able to look after her household, the local authority is required to provide assistance. Such "home helps" come periodically to perform such tasks as looking after children, doing the cooking, cleaning, etc. These services were developed chiefly for those women temporarily incapacitated by physical illness who were being treated in their own homes. The service is also available to mental patients residing at home who are not yet able to resume the full burdens of housekeeping and household management.

"Meals on Wheels"

As part of an overall program to maintain as many elderly people as possible in the community, the local authority provides a service staffed largely by volunteers, bringing hot meals to the homes of aged individuals unable to prepare food for themselves. While these aged people are not necessarily mentally ill, if it were not for programs such as "Meals on Wheels" many of them would have to be cared for in institutions. This service reduces the demand for mental hospital beds.

VOLUNTARY AGENCIES

A wide variety of voluntary agencies dealing with problems of mental health is found throughout England (64, 86). Some are small and purely local; others are quite large and national in scope. Many are entirely independent, supported completely from voluntary contributions. Others are quasi-official agencies receiving some public support in addition to funds raised in a voluntary manner.

Councils of Social Services

Most areas are served by Councils of Social Services: voluntary social agencies partly subsidized by the local authorities, usually with local authority officials represented on the managing boards (86). These agencies provide the traditional case work and other social aid services. In London, they support an institution not known in most of the United States, called the Citizens' Advice Bureaux.

The Citizens' Advice Bureaux (CABs)

(CABs) are specialized agencies, coordinated by a National Citizens' Advice Bureau Council, with around 500 offices throughout the country. The pattern of their distribution varies from place to place. In London there are usually a number of them within each local authority area, staffed either by professional social workers, volunteers, or both. They are available to anyone who wishes to come in for advice about problems of any sort. The type of work they do varies with the neighborhood in which they are located. In some neighborhoods people need assistance with practical, everyday problems of living or in dealing with the official hierarchy of the local or central government. Sometimes legal assistance is required, sometimes assistance in finding housing. Sometimes general information is sought, and sometimes the client comes in merely to talk to someone.

The Citizens' Advice Bureaux probably represent a major force in primary prevention of mental illness. They provide a receptive ear for those who have no one else to talk to, allowing people to let off steam who otherwise might become seriously troubled and perhaps disturbed. By giving advice and assistance to those requiring help in coping with problems of daily living, housing, welfare, neighborhood problems, etc., it is likely that they serve to forestall the development of internal stress which would otherwise lead to decompensation. The workers can often recognize early manifestations of mental illness in the clients and may help the client recognize his need for psychiatric treatment. Some of the functions of the Citizens' Advice Bureaux have been emulated by the various neighborhood service centers established in the United States as part of the primary prevention programs of the community mental health services.

National Association of Mental Health

This is a national voluntary organization comparable to its counterpart in the United States. Local chapters are to be found throughout Britain. A major service provided by this organization is to disseminate information, chiefly to the public, about problems of mental illness. It is also a forceful lobby towards the betterment of conditions and facilities for the mentally ill. In addition, a number of local branches provide community facilities for former mental patients. An example is represented by the activities of the Camden Association for Mental Health, which provides group activities, several social clubs, and meeting facilities for programs conducted by other groups.

Special-Problem Organizations

Voluntary organizations have been developed to deal with specific aspects of mental health problems. Some of these are sponsored by private groups interested in helping their fellow man; others are self-help groups; still others are specialized, providing facilities to cope with particular problems.

The Samaritans is an organization founded by a clergyman to help those contemplating suicide. They operate in a manner similar to comparable suicide prevention organizations in the United States. The Blackfriars is a group dedicated to helping those released from prison or picked up as vagabonds or potential delinquents. The Rudolf Steiner organization operates a network of "schools" for mentally ill children geared for treatment of those quite severely disturbed. While these schools are operated under private auspices, children are referred, and payment for the treatment is usually underwritten by the local authorities. Alcoholics Anonymous and Synanon are self-help programs for alcoholics and drug addicts identical with their counterparts in the United States. The Mental After-Care Association and the Richmond Fellowship operate hostels in the community as sheltered living accommodations for former patients in mental hospitals.

Hospital Volunteers

Most mental hospitals utilize the services of volunteers. Some volunteers serve as individuals; others are organized in groups such as the League of Friends. Some contribute financial help for amenities that otherwise would be unavailable to patients. Some serve as visitors to patients who have no family. Still others become interested in particular patients as a kind of "big brother," generally on the basis of some common interest. They may take patients from the hospital for outings, give assistance in finding employment, etc. Other groups provide special activities or treats for the patients in the hospitals.

The parents of the mentally subnormal have a rather strong and active organization which serves both as a lobbying group and as a provider of direct services for the mentally subnormal.

PART TWO: THE MENTAL HEALTH PROGRAMS

"Oh wad some power the giftie gie us
To see oursels as others see us!"

Robert Burns

Part II is arranged to illustrate the types of mental health programs discussed in more general terms in Part I. The programs described are examples of successful approaches to community mental health services. As previously mentioned, the success of a given program has resulted, in most instances, from the efforts of a particular person, and the program itself usually experienced some deterioration if he moved to another post. None of the programs is a "typical" one, nor is my coverage of health facilities intended to be comprehensive.

I have arranged the programs as follows: programs operated by the mental hospitals, programs operated by the local authorities (communities), programs involving the cooperation of the mental hospital and the local authority (referred to as "joint programs"), and mental health programs within the setting of a general hospital. In addition, I have included a chapter on voluntary services and one covering three unique programs: The Tavistock Centre, the Institute of Family Psychiatry, and the Insitute of Psychiatry and the Maudsley Hospital, London. For in-depth study I have chosen the programs related to community mental health services in Camden Borough, London.

At the time of my first visit in 1969, community mental health services in England had developed primarily through evolutionary changes. By 1971, the recommednations of the Seebohm Report (Report of the Committee on Local Authority and Allied Personal Social Services) were being implemented, and the mental health programs were undergoing far-reaching alterations. I should like to emphasize that the impact of the Seebohm Report was greatest on those programs where the local authority was the main provider of mental health services. In programs operated mainly by the mental hospitals, where local authority services had been minimal, the changes brought about by Seebohm were less evident.

The descriptions of hospitals in terms of architecture, general organization, number of staff members, and types of activities are based on my personal observations. I have had to add to or modify some of my original impressions to depict the changes occurring between 1969 and the time of my follow-up visit in 1971. Additional modifications concerning current and anticipated changes within the health service are based on discussions with mental health experts in England and correspondence subsequent to 1971.

None of my English friends whose programs are described in the following pages will be totally satisfied with the account of his particular endeavor. Some errors of omission or commission undoubtedly reflect the author's fallibility; others may result from the fact that subsequent developments have rendered my observations obsolete. Not infrequently, what may appear to the protagonists as discrepancies will be traceable to the unique vantage points from which we inevitably view ourselves and others.

For any errors of fact, I apologize. For differences in point of view and emphasis, I take full responsibility. In the last analysis, these reports represent one American psychiatrist's perception of what he observed in England.

7

Programs operated by the mental hospitals

The hospital-operated programs represent the attempt of the mental hospitals to provide community care for discharged patients in situations where local authority facilities are minimal or absent, or where cooperative work with local authority groups has not been feasible.

In 1959, eleven years after the mental hospitals were brought under the National Health Service, the clinical and administrative responsibilities formerly vested in the medical superintendent were redelegated (78). Administration of both mental and general hospitals became the responsibility of hospital management committees, which generally oversee the operation of groups of hospitals. Supervision of clinical activities within the mental hospitals became the province of one or more consultant psychiatrists. Typically, the hospital is divided into several clinical "firms," each staffed by a team of psychiatrists of various grades headed by a senior consultant. In some instances, a marked difference in philosophy exists between senior consultants at the same hospital, so that within a single institution, programs which differ radically from each other in conception and implementation coexist side by side. Such is the case at Littlemore Hospital, Oxford and, to a much lesser extent, at the Graylingwell Hospital, Chichester, both of which are described below.

GRAYLINGWELL HOSPITAL

Located just outside of Chichester, in the county of Sussex, Graylingwell Hospital is close to the southern English coastal resort area. The old Victorian buildings of the hospital are situated on attractive grounds. There are presently 1,000 beds at Graylingwell to provide for a rather large catchment area extending from the city of Chichester to the city of Worthing, 20 miles away, with a total population of approximately 280,000.

Dr. Joshua Carse was physician superintendent of Graylingwell when he conducted the well known "Worthing Experiment" (10, 11, 12). As a means of reducing overcrowding at the hospital, Dr. Carse's experiment was aimed at treating as many patients as possible in their own homes. The psychiatrist made repeated domiciliary visits and advised relatives on care and management problems. In this way, Carse was able to reduce hospital admissions by 59% and to demonstrate that these patients could be maintained at home (10, 11, 12). This initial effort at community psychiatric care established the hospital's responsibility in the area. Since the local health authority did not participate in the experiment, the relationship between the hospital and the local authority has remained minimal over the years.

In addition to Graylingwell Hospital, the Acre, a day hospital established by Carse and located in Worthing, is operated by a treatment team from Graylingwell. There is also a new day hospital, Kingsmead, on the Graylingwell campus. In addition, outpatient clinics are conducted in general hospitals in Chichester and Bognor. A psychiatric inpatient unit is planned for the Worthing General Hospital, but there are no general hospital psychiatric beds there at present.

At the time of my visit, the staff at Graylingwell consisted of three psychiatric consultants, three social workers, one medical assistant, two psychologists, two senior registrars, two ordinary registrars, and two clinical assistants. The hospital contains an acute admission ward, rehabilitation wards, an Alcoholic Unit, and a 36-bed geriatric ward. There is also a "Social Therapy Unit" and a "Psychotherapy Unit" ("closed for redecoration" at the time of my visit). The latter is primarily used for relatively short-stay patients who are treated with group psychotherapy. The Alcoholic Unit also emphasizes group therapy and is closely linked with the community Alcoholics Ananymous program, which maintains contact with patients discharged from the unit.

The acute-admission ward caters to 31 patients, mostly short-stay (4–6 weeks). Some stay only a few days. There are two dormitories, one for patients requiring close observation and one for patients who do not. The ward staff consists of three nurses in the morning, three in the afternoon, and two at night.

Major interest and emphasis at the hospital centers on two rehabilitation wards where chronic patients are sent in preparation for discharge from the hospital. The rehabilitation wards, one for men and one for women, are operated in conjunction with the hospital's Industrial Therapy Unit.

The Industrial Therapy Unit

In 1966, Graylingwell Hospital opened its Industrial Therapy Unit. A few patients come to the unit from the community, having been previously discharged from the hospital. The bulk of the patients, however, are inpatients, particularly from the rehabilitation wards, but also from throughout the hospital. The patients' length of stay in the unit varies. There is no time limit; they remain until they are able to go to work or return home, or until the staff feels that it would be more beneficial for them to be placed on another unit. A few of the patients have been there continuously since the unit opened; others had formerly gone out to jobs, but returned to the unit when their community adjustment faltered. A total of 200 patients work in the unit, 80 of whom are from the rehabilitation wards. A few former patients, now living in the community, use the industrial therapy activities as a sort of day program.

The patients are assessed and reassessed during their stay on the Industrial Therapy Unit. Dr. Norman Capstick, the psychiatric consultant in charge of this program, states that "assessment is therapy and therapy is assessment." Assessments are recorded on charts which indicate work skills as well as personality factors. When a new patient arrives, a work report is prepared by five staff members. Five evaluations are made within the patient's first six weeks on the unit, and a re-evaluation is made when it is thought necessary—usually between two and three weeks, but sometimes as long as six months later. Between assessments, patients are closely observed for changes by members of the staff. In addition to the work evaluations, the Wittenborn Scale has been used for personality assessment. At the time of my visit a new scale was being constructed by a psychology student at the hospital. The patient's assessments are regularly discussed at staff meetings.

The unit is run along the lines of a factory. Patients clock in and out. They are graded according to their work capacities, skills, and reliability into five or six grades and are paid by the hour according to their grade. A board is kept in the office giving details about each patient on the unit, such as his age, name, and place of work. For discharged patients living in the community, the place of residence is also noted. These details are recorded for two years after discharge.

The weekly payroll for the Industrial Therapy Unit is roughly £200. Patients in the lowest grade receive 25 new pence, those in the highest, £2.00 per week; the average rate is approximately £1.00. During 1968–69 the unit received £10,000 for their work, £8,000 of which was paid to the patients; the remainder was utilized to upgrade the facilities of the unit. There is a steady flow of work from various commercial and industrial enterprises. Most of it is handwork, but some activities require power tools, bench drills, and heat solder. This special equipment is supplied by the industrial firm requiring the particular process.

About ten activities go on simultaneously. The standard of work is high, at least the equivalent of standards of commercial shops. The unit even does some work for export which is of such high caliber that it leaves the unit already packed for shipment out of the country. Occasionally rush jobs are done for the industrial firms.

The type of work performed on the ITU includes sub-assembly of small plastic parts, packing of sterile dressings (this consists of stamping packets, putting in the contents, and heat-sealing the packets prior to sterilization), stamping of all doctors' prescription pads in the area (a job done mostly by old women), assembling wooden toys, and even inspecting of plastic work performed by commercial industrial firms.

Patients normally work five hours a day, although some of the more active ones work seven hours. Most of the patients are on tranquilizing medication of some kind, and a number also receive anti-Parkinsonian drugs. A group of 45-50 patients from the locked wards also work in the unit in a special group. Their activities include assembling toys of various kinds (blackboards or deck chairs), assembling plastic oil containers, and disassembling obsolete telephone equipment. There is also an assembly-line job making hat stands. A group of regressed patients hacks scraps of wood into firewood kindling, which is bundled and sold.

The simpler tasks are assigned to the less effective patients in the lowest grade. Some patients from the highest grade are assigned to check the work of the others. Such assignments carry considerable status and create incentives for the patients even beyond that provided by the payment scheme.

The unit has grown considerably since it was started, and its facilities have been extended beyond the walls of the building in which it was originally housed. According to Dr. Capstick, a new extension onto the original building was constructed by staff and patients to serve as a storeroom and to provide additional work space, and a new welding shop has been added. Some of the old farm buildings which had fallen into disrepair when the hospital's agricultural program was abandoned some years ago have been rehabilitated by nursing staff and patients. Here a greenhouse has been built where patients raise plants in seed boxes they have made themselves. The patients sell both plants and seed boxes in the community. They also maintain a garden where they grow fruit and vegetables for sale in the town. Here also the patients make decorative concrete tiles for garden walls. The tiles are formed into designs created by the patients, who are even experimenting with new types of concrete slab especially suited for gardens. Another workshop in the farm buildings houses 30-40 patients who check commercially manufactured plastic bottles, reject the defective ones, and pack the others.

The full-time staff of the Industrial Therapy Unit consists of the director, Miss Platt, a mental nurse with a major interest in rehabilitation, two staff nurses, and two carpenters. There is a part-time gardener as well as various other part-time staff.

The Social Therapy Unit

The Social Therapy Unit is run by Mrs. E. Kirby, a former film actress who also operates a sheltered living accommodation in Chichester for former inpatients (Kirby House). The unit has facilities for 45 patients, the usual attendance being 35. The patients, of both sexes and from various wards of the hospital, come voluntarily. Nurses sometimes accompany locked-ward patients who wish to participate in the social therapy program. The schedule on the unit is much less rigid than that of the other areas of the hospital.

Social therapy activities, generally quite unstructured, include country dancing, cooking, and bingo. Patients play cards and table tennis, listen to records, and participate in drama groups and play-reading sessions. Aged patients play musical chairs. Once a week there are free discussion groups. Some activities are conducted in the evenings. There is a social on Friday evening and also on Saturday morning. Outings are arranged to places of interest, and patients also engage in inter-hospital sports, chiefly cricket and football. A patients' committee makes up the programs and selects groups of patients to conduct their own activities, such as teaching drama and music, giving informal talks, and conducting musical evenings. Except for the discussion groups, which have closed membership, any patient who wishes may drop in and participate in any activity he chooses.

Sheltered living accommodations in the community provide places for discharged patients. As previously mentioned, Kirby House, a supervised hostel operated privately by the "social therapist," houses eight patients who look after themselves and pay their own way. Selbourne House, a small house in the community, and "Cortus Avenue," a pair of council houses, are run by the patients without supervision. Some discharged patients go to nursing homes where they both live and work. The practice, initiated by Dr. Carse, of making multiple home visits to patients residing in the community continues to be carried out by the present consultants, although on a smaller scale.

A major problem at the hospital has been the geriatric population, because so many aged people come to the seaside resorts, and hence into the catchment area, to retire. Dr. Capstick does not feel that geriatrics is a proper problem for a mental hospital, preferring instead to establish specialized hospitals for the aged, which contain psychogeriatric units.

Much volunteer work goes on at Graylingwell Hospital. Volunteer townspeople may be found assisting in the wards, helping at meal times, making beds, running a band, or giving art or music lessons. A Townsmen's Guild in the hospital establishes a liaison with patients prior to their discharge, so that when they leave the hospital they are already members of an organization. Women volunteers often take patients out for the day or run theater parties for them at the renowned Chichester Playhouse. In nearby Littlehampton a volunteer group helps to introduce discharged chronic patients to members of the community who may be of help to them. The Littlehampton community assists ex-patients in a number of ways and encourages former patients to contribute to the community through such services as pushing invalids in wheelchairs, changing library books for the aged, and walking dogs. The philosophy is that a patient who has received help in the past is obligated to help others. Foulbourne, a nearby hospital, has a voluntary organization called the "Backbenchers." Every two or three months the hospital arranges a teaparty for these volunteers, and in return the "Backbenchers" take patients on outings, help in the wards, or perform other services.

Local people assist in other ways, too. For example, people in various trades or professions will acquaint themselves with patients who had been in the same fields and visit them in the hospital. They can then discuss matters of mutual interest, making the visit more meaningful, and the townsperson can facilitate the patient's return to constructive employment after he leaves the hospital. The hospital conducts public education programs to gain the attention of the townspeople and to enlist the aid of the community in behalf of the patients. The local Citizens' Advice Bureau has been asked to set up an office at the hospital to help patients who have been out of touch with the community to learn about community services and facilities. However, the relationship with the local authority has not been good. This extended even to the mental welfare officer, who refused to visit the hospital, had little knowledge of discharged patients, and therefore took little part in aftercare programs. Dr. Capstick believes that the local authorities should provide facilities for mental defectives and geriatric patients, but is satisfied to have the hospital conduct the community programs for the mentally ill.

The relationship with the local authority improved somewhat when three social workers from the staff at Graylingwell, experienced in their field and well-known to the hospital, transferred to the local authority and assumed the roles of MWOs. Since the implementation of the Seebohm Report, which created a new Social Service Department, there has been further deterioration in hospital-community relations. The MWO responsibility has now been distributed among the many social workers of the new Social Service Department, most of whom have neither experience with nor interest in psychiatric problems. In addition, the publicity that the Social Service Department received in the community, as a result of Seebohm, temporarily increased the workload of the department and further impaired its efficiency.

Kingsmead, a day hospital located on the Graylingwell grounds, was opened in January 1969. It is run by a senior consultant (other than Dr. Capstick) and serves only the local Chichester portion of the catchment area. Patients come by their own transportation or are brought by local authority ambulances. The unit occupies a rehabilitated old house and contains a sizeable occupational therapy room, a kitchen, a dining room, and day rooms. While Kingsmead is supposed to be separate from Graylingwell proper, it is still attached in many ways to the main hospital which, for example, provides the lunches for the patients. A number of therapeutic activities are conducted. Electroconvulsive therapy is given twice a week; some patients with phobias are treated with behavior therapy; and there is extensive use of occupational therapy. There are regular group therapy meetings but no individual psychotherapy.

Graylingwell Hospital also houses an important unit of the Medical Research Council devoted to study and evaluation of community mental health programs, and noted elsewhere in this report.

LITTLEMORE HOSPITAL

Littlemore Hospital, Oxford, was built in 1846, and serves a huge catchment area of 400,000 population, including the city of Oxford and surrounding districts (112). The hospital's function is divided into two distinct clinical divisions. At the head of one is Dr. John Duffield, and Dr. F. J. J. Letemendia works with him. Dr. B. M. Mandelbrote heads the other, assisted by Dr. B. Pomryn. Each division is autonomous and quite distinct in character from the other.

Rivalry between the two divisions produces occasional friction between them, although all four consultants maintain communication with one another through regularly scheduled meetings. The principal nursing officer of the hospital supervises nursing activities of both divisions, while the social workers and occupational therapists are linked with particular teams. Disagreement between the teams of consultants about managing the patients has led to partisanship on this issue by members of the administrative staff, who find the conventional approach of one team less disturbing to the administrative equilibrium than the experimental approach followed by the other.

The division of Duffield and Letemendia functions in a rather traditional institutional pattern; that is, it is organized into wards for acute and chronic patients; sexes are separate, and staff are in uniform. Duffield, who has been at the hospital since 1945, spends most of his time in outpatient activity and in making domiciliary visits. Some parts of his unit have been physically remodelled and are therefore in good condition and attractive. The level of medical management is quite good for acute patients, resembling somewhat the approach of a psychiatric unit in a general hospital. Long-stay patients, however, are usually treated custodially and are managed chiefly by the nursing staff.

The division of Mandelbrote and Pomryn is more modern and inventive. When Mandelbrote arrived in 1959, the total hospital population was 940, equally divided between the two divisions. The present inpatient population is 460, of which only 165 reside in Mandelbrote's division, which has been more successful than the other in reducing the inpatient population. On his arrival, Mandelbrote introduced the therapeutic-community approach, organizing the clinical program into four "communities" within the hospital. Each community contains sufficient ward area to house its resident patients, but there are no organizations along ward lines. Instead, the communities are the living settings, intended to provide for the personal and social needs of the patients. Sexes of both staff and patients are mixed and staff are not in uniform. In each community the therapeutic milieu varies according to the kind of patient resident in the community, and each community has a name: Ashhurst, Phoenix, Mayo, and Isis. Each unit is fairly autonomous, although all are under the same two consultants, Mandelbrote and Pomryn, who evaluate the patients referred for hospitalization and decide which unit they will be admitted to.

The Ashhurst Clinic

The Ashhurst Clinic started as a 54-bed insulin clinic serving the entire hospital. This unit is now divided into two parts, one for each of the two clinical divisions. Mandelbrote's part serves as a mental health center for people with suitable homes and employment, who can be treated on an inpatient basis with group psychotherapy. In addition, there are also several therapeutic groups for day patients and outpatients linked with the Ashhurst Clinic. In Ashhurst, as in each of the other units in Mandelbrote's division, there is a continuity-of-care program; the same staff looks after the common group of patients regardless of whether their status happens to be inpatient, outpatient, or day-hospital patient.

In Mandelbrote's portion of Ashhurst there are facilities for 25 inpatients and 40-60 day patients. Some of the day patients attend five days per week, others attend anywhere from one to four days, so that the number of day patients on the unit at any given time will vary. Because of the intensity and effectiveness of the therapeutic program, the need for inpatient beds at the Ashhurst had declined to the point where, at the time of my first visit, there was only one inpatient hospitalized on the unit; the remainder were day patients. Since that time, Ashhurst has continued to operate on a day-patient basis, and now there are no inpatients in Mandelbrote's division.

Ashhurst is supervised by a senior registrar, assisted by two part-time clinical assistants who are employed under a special program for bringing married women doctors into the Health Service on a part-time basis. At the time of my visit, the senior registrar had just returned from Dr. Gerald Caplan's program at Harvard University, Boston, with many new and provocative ideas and was leading the staff in discussions involving a rethinking of their therapeutic concepts. Consequently, Ashhurst's function was undergoing a change. According to Mandelbrote, the new emphasis is on using nurses in the community, and a member of the nursing staff is now attached part-time to a family doctor practice.

Ashhurst also serves as a meeting place for MWOs, health officers, and general practitioners. There are two old MWOs without social work training, and three trained social workers serving as MWOs employed by the local authority. The table of organization calls for as many as six qualified social workers to be employed by the hospital as a whole, three assigned to each of the two clinical divisions; they do not have that many actually on the staff, however. Every Monday morning the hospital social workers and the local authority MWOs meet with the doctors and the rehabilitation officer of the hospital, whose function is similar to that of the Disablement Resettlement Officer of the Department of Employment and Productivity, formerly the Ministry of Labour. The hospital rehabilitation officer is highly regarded. Well trained, he supervises the industrial therapy programs of the hospital and also participates in the efforts at placing patients in employment situations. At the Monday morning meeting, all admissions and discharges of the past week are discussed and assignments of patients to social workers are made. These include assignment of patients to the MWOs, who function in this connection as if they were hospital social workers. Following the implementation of the White Paper on April 1, 1974, the hospital social workers at Littlemore will be absorbed into the Local Authority Social Service Department.

Twelve months following the patient's discharge, a follow-up conference is held, prior to which each patient is seen by the assigned social worker, and a report made. This report is discussed at the follow-up conference to evaluate the patient's community adjustment and to take the next necessary therapeutic measures.

The Phoenix Unit

The Phoenix Unit, opened in 1961, is based on large-community therapy, in contrast to the Ashhurst, which is based on small communities. In the Phoenix Unit the patient group meets as a whole in conferences, similar to therapeutic community conferences, daily at 8:30 A.M. In addition, there are two further sessions, one held in the evening for those who work during the day, the other a session for relatives of patients being treated in the Phoenix Unit. Additional meetings are held on an *ad hoc* basis if a crisis develops. Meetings are led by a patient-chairman, and a patient-secretary keeps the minutes. These meetings deal with personal problems and psychodynamics of the patients, in addition to the patients' common problems of daily living on the unit and problems of tolerance in the community. A psychiatrist supervises each of the meetings. The Phoenix Unit is supervised by a senior registrar assisted by a junior registrar and a senior house officer. However, Mandelbrote takes one of these meetings each week, and Pomryn three. Each meeting is followed by a discussion for teaching purposes, which is attended by a patient-management group.

Since the Phoenix Unit started, 120 long-stay patients of the hospital have been members. Of these, 90% have been sent out of the hospital into the community, and 10% have remained in the hospital throughout this time. Ten per cent of those patients sent into the community have returned as inpatients. Diagnostic categories include the most difficult patients. Many of the Phoenix Unit patients are chronic institutionalized schizophrenics considered to be candidates for rehabilitation. In addition to schizophrenia, patients suffer from other psychoses associated with acute behavioral disturbances, and there are a few with long-standing character disorders. Patients with severe personality disorders and chronic schizophrenic patients are usually admitted directly to the Phoenix Unit. Patients who are acutely ill, with suitable family situations and strong community ties, are usually admitted to the Ashhurst Unit.

Patients with serious legal problems, including prisoners suffering from mental disorders, may be admitted to Littlemore, in which case they too usually are admitted to the Phoenix Unit. The prison (Gremdon Underwood) has a psychiatric unit which, however, does not usually admit psychopaths. In addition, there are hospitals for the criminally insane, such as Broadmoor. These hospitals, as well as the prison psychiatric unit, sometimes send their staff to the Phoenix Unit for training.

It is difficult to evaluate the effectiveness of the Phoenix Unit. The type of patient, as well as the type of therapeutic approach, tends to arouse the hostility of the Littlemore administrative staff (excepting of course those staff members actually working on the Phoenix Unit itself). Sometimes the patients create such havoc or damage that they have to be sent off to prisons. For example, one severely psychopathic patient, who was admitted with his wife as a family to the Phoenix Unit, spent two years there making trouble the entire time. Finally he forged a prescription to get drugs, was picked up by the police, and sent to prison. His wife went to live in Oxford, and when the patient was released from prison he joined her. He has not been in trouble in the two years since leaving prison; at least he hasn't been picked up by the police during this time. Mandelbrote feels that while the patient did not do well during the period he spent on the Phoenix Unit itself, his experience on the unit formed the basis for his later satisfactory community adjustment.

On the Phoenix Unit there is one outstanding occupational therapist whose knowledge of psychodynamics and whose ability with patients is superior even to that of the social workers. Other occupational therapists are more traditionally group oriented. There is only one industrial therapy unit for the entire hospital, but, in Mandelbrote's division, industrial therapy projects tend to be farmed out to the respective units according to their nature and complexity, and according to the type of patient there.

The Mayo Unit

The most "damaged patients" under the age of 75 who are not physically ill are absorbed by the Mayo Unit. Originally the residents of this unit were a group of approximately 30 young women, often mute, incontinent, and very regressed. Many have brain damage, general paresis, or other organic pathology. These patients were successfully managed by a training regime, and then a group of similar male patients was added. The Mayo Unit is now a mixed community run similarly to the Phoenix Unit, but giving greater attention to personal habits and appearance. As the overall approach has been fairly successful, responsibilities given to the patients have gradually been increased. The Mayo Unit is supervised by Dr. Peter Aqulnik, a medical assistant. In addition to the inpatients, a small day-patient complement made up of discharged former inpatients live in group homes in the community. Some of these patients had been in sheltered workshops. When I visited, there were eight nurses on duty for each shift, representing the highest number of nurses ever at the Mayo Unit.

On the Mayo Unit there is a therapeutic community meeting each morning, followed by a staff discussion. Small groups of patients attend this meeting, along with the staff, and discuss the assessment of their progress in interpersonal and work areas. Afterwards, the patients are divided into work groups and are assigned to a variety of projects, such as occupational therapy activities and industrial therapy projects, particularly the dismantling of obsolete telephones. After 4:00 P.M. there is a range of social activities for the patients. Recreational activities, including occasional outings, are likewise planned for them.

Many volunteers, affiliated with groups such as "The League of Friends," help the Mayo Unit. These volunteers also organize outings and social activities, such as the "day fete" I observed during my visit.

At one time the Mayo Unit housed up to 80 patients; the census on the day of my visit was 48, ten of whom were living in a hostel arrangement in the hospital. No nurse is assigned to this group. The nurses on the Mayo Unit are assigned according to the degree of patient need. Patients admitted directly to the Mayo Unit include those with severe head injuries, epilepsy, and central nervous system disorders. An aged regressed schizophrenic may be admitted, but rarely.

The Isis Unit

Here reside the aged and the physically ill patients. Part of the unit contains a "sick unit" of twenty-eight beds shared equally between the two divisions. These beds are used for patients with acute physical illness. When the patient has recovered from the somatic illness, he returns to his home ward in the respective division of the hospital whence he came. The sick unit is also used for drug and alcohol withdrawals.

The Isis Unit also contains fifty old people of both sexes, in addition to another group of twenty-five very frail and debilitated people of both sexes who are treated separately with habit training. These are severely demented and incontinent patients and include the hard core geriatric population. Occasionally some of the patients requiring specialized habit-training can be gradually absorbed into the Isis Unit proper.

The two divisions of the hospital share the nursing staff equally. In Mandelbrote's division 90 nurses serve 175 patients, including the 10 patients from the other division who are being treated on the sick unit. None of the nurses wear uniforms, nor do the occupational therapists or any of the other staff. Mandelbrote states that "Littlemore has the best nursing staff in the country."

Hostels, Group Homes, and Other Related Services

In addition to her inpatient responsibilities, one nurse serves as coordinator of the hostels and group homes in the community. There are two supervised hostels, which were initiated by Mandelbrote in 1960 based upon his prior experience with hostels. At the time of my visit, one of the hostels lacked a warden; the other was fully staffed. A "home group" is a patient work group of five or six people living in a group home, an accommodation for former inpatients, unsupervised, although a student volunteer often helps to get the home started. Eleven group homes serve both divisions of the hospital. Most of the resident patients come from the Phoenix Unit, although some are from the Mayo or Isis units.

Each unit has its own day-patient groups, consisting usually of former inpatients, although some are admitted directly as day patients. The nature of the patient's problems determines which unit he will be assigned to. Once he is assigned to a particular unit, he receives continued care. Ashhurst carries approximately 20 day-patients per day although its potential number of patients is 50. As previously noted, at the time of my visit there was only one inpatient in Ashhurst. The day-patient population on the Phoenix Unit is likewise around 20. The Mayo Unit has 12 day patients, the Isis Unit 17. Thus a total of up to 80 day patients per day attend programs in the various units of this division.

The outpatient services are organized according to the particular consultant in charge, rather than according to the two clinical divisions which characterize the inpatient services. At Whitney, fourteen miles from Oxford, a group of doctors work at a center which includes an MOH and consultants in several disciplines, including three psychiatrists. This serves as a base for one of the major outpatient clinics where Mandelbrote works. Mandelbrote also conducts another fortnightly outpatient clinic at Chipping-Norton.

Mandelbrote and his division are also involved in other community-based activities. A new drug-dependency unit was opened in August 1970, as a regional service to provide continuity of care between hospital and community regarding programs of drug and alcohol abuse. In addition to the community facilities, there are facilities for inpatient treatment of drug-dependent patients and alcoholics.

The Isis Centre

According to Mandelbrote, a special community clinic in Oxford was opened in November 1970, known as the Isis Centre. It is directed by a consultant psychiatrist and staffed by a team of doctors, nurses, social workers, and occupational therapists. It serves as a walk-in clinic, crisis intervention service, and information center. New clients are seen by whichever staff member is available, and interviews are kept as informal as possible. Initially, no attempt is made to take notes or fill out forms; instead the interviewer tries to establish a relationship with the client, understand his problem, and explain the setup of the Isis Centre. Following the interview, the staff member reports the case to the rest of the team, which meets twice a week. After discussing the case, the team makes suggestions on how to provide help for the client. They may refer him for a psychiatric examination, possibly with admission to a hospital, or they may arrange for group therapy. In some cases, individual counseling or supportive psychotherapy or both are recommended. Many people who may need some help, but not necessarily full-scale psychiatric treatment, can benefit from such facilities as the Isis Centre, which in these instances assumes a preventive role.

The Isis Centre also functions as an educational facility for people in the caring professions, such as health visitors, teachers, counselors in various social fields, probation officers, etc., enabling them to cope with emotional problems encountered in their work. There are sensitivity groups for primary school teachers, and in the future others in the caring professions will also participate in such encounter groups.

Littlemore Hospital is affiliated with the medical school at Oxford, and recently the hospital's participation in the medical education program has increased. At the present time there are two months of full-time undergraduate training in psychiatry, and many students spend approximately six months at Littlemore Hospital.

MARLBOROUGH DAY HOSPITAL

The Marlborough Day Hospital was founded in 1946 by Dr. Joshua Bierer and, together with one in Montreal set up by Dr. Ewen Cameron, it was the first of its kind in the world (5). It was originally established to fulfill the social and therapeutic needs of patients who did not require inpatient treatment but were, nevertheless, incapacitated by psychiatric illness (26). In 1949 the program was taken over by the National Health Service, and it moved to the present premises. Located in a pleasant part of northwest London (St. Johns Wood), the hospital now occupies an old house. The occupational therapy unit and an inpatient unit are in another old house, formerly the home of Thomas Huxley, behind the main building. The day hospital is not connected with any other institution nor does it serve a particular catchment area, but it is administratively a part of the St. Charles Hospital management group which supplies all dry goods, stores, linen, drugs, etc., and also provides the midday meals for the patients.

The staff consists of 4 registrars, 2 clinical psychologists, 2 full-time nurses and 16 part-time nursing staff, 1 part-time speech therapist, and 3 psychiatric social workers. In addition, several consultants make weekly visits to the day hospital. Although many of the staff members, including all of the occupational therapists and social workers, are employed full time, part-time help is extensively used.

Patients are referred by general practitioners, mental hospitals, teaching hospitals, and social agencies. The hospital is not especially selective regarding admissions, but does not normally accept acutely violent or aggressive patients. Around a third of the patient population suffer from various forms of schizophrenia, a third from psychoneuroses, and a third have various character and personality disorders. Aged patients are sometimes accepted, but the staff believes that such patients would be better cared for in the Borough Occupation Center or in special geriatric centers. Approximately one-third of the patients remain at the Marlborough Day Hospital between six weeks and three months. Another third remain three to nine months, and one third attend longer than nine months. Former patients may be readmitted for brief periods if necessary. Most patients discharged from the day hospital continue to attend the outpatient clinic, and many participate in the therapeutic social clubs as well.

Approximately 30-40 patients attend every day between the hours of 9:30 A.M. and 4:00 P.M. The regular weekly program consists of occupational therapy, group meetings, art classes, drama classes, outings, etc. Some patients are members of small closed therapeutic groups; about half receive fairly intensive individual psychotherapy. Electroconvulsive therapy (ECT) is also administered in selected cases. At the time of my first visit, four patients were receiving ECT, all of them inpatients. ECT is not given on an outpatient basis.

Most of the patients' time is spent in the occupational therapy unit. The unit is well equipped, enabling patients to participate in a variety of activities. The unit has a kitchen used for teaching elementary cookery and also for preparing the morning tea, around which a patient discussion group has developed.

Since Marlborough Day Hospital does not yet serve a defined catchment area, patients may come from considerable distances to attend. As the patients' travel time ranges between fifteen minutes to an hour each way, the staff does not always "chase" those who sometimes do not turn up. Recently, more and more of the patients come from Westminster or the neighboring borough, rather than from greater distances.

A patient referred to the day hospital will first be interviewed by one of the consultants and then scheduled to attend a meeting of the Admissions Committee, held regularly at 3:00 P.M. Wednesdays. There he meets various members of the staff representing the different professional disciplines. After the committee meeting, the prospective patient is introduced to the other day hospital patients at afternoon tea and then invited to attend the next morning. This procedure serves both to screen prospective admissions in order that unsuitable patients not be admitted and also facilitates the introduction of new patients into the group. The Admissions Committee looks for some degree of motivation to attend with the intention of improvement, and is likely to exclude acutely disturbed or overtly psychotic patients.

The active outpatient-service admits approximately 500 new cases a year. Most patients receive individual psychotherapy on a once-a-week basis, and in addition there are six closed therapy groups. Many patients referred to Marlborough Day Hospital are admitted directly to the outpatient service rather than to the day hospital, whereas other patients have spent a period of time as day patients before being seen as outpatients.

An unusual feature of the Marlborough Day Hospital is the child psychiatry facilities. A child guidance unit for children who are highly emotionally disturbed operates twice weekly under the direction of a child psychiatrist, assisted by a social worker and psychologist. The unit is not directly connected with the Education Department, and therefore is unique, being completely under medical auspices. However, an educational psychologist from the Education Department makes a weekly visit. There is no special clinic for adolescents, although there are outpatient therapy groups especially for adolescent members.

In addition, a small day-treatment unit for autistic children operates Monday through Thursday. The unit is under the direction of a trained child psychotherapist, but is staffed chiefly by women volunteers. The unit is run on a one patient to one "aunt" ratio. On an average day, there are usually ten to twelve patients ranging in age from five to twelve years. Although the "aunts" are volunteers, it is essential that they attend regularly in order that a therapeutic relationship can be established between patient and aunt. If either the aunt or the child is absent for any length of time, the child tends to regress. Most patients receive no medication. When the children reach the age of 12, they must leave the unit; most are sent to special schools, such as those operated by the Rudolph Steiner Organization. The Parents' Autistic Society has also organized a special school at Ealing for such children.

Marlborough Day Hospital engages in a number of teaching activities for psychiatric nurses, social work students, occupational therapy students, probation officers, and teachers, giving postgraduate courses for general practitioners from time to time. The teaching program also includes undergraduate teaching for medical students from the Royal Free Hospital, who attend in groups of two or three on a one-day-per-week basis for a period of a month.

As originally set up by Dr. Bierer, the Marlborough Day Hospital was unique in being independent of any other institution, and in not serving a specific catchment area. In addition to the day program, Bierer inaugurated a service whereby the day patients might be kept in the hospital overnight, if a particular need for doing so might arise. Bierer's approach with his patients was quite permissive; one of the basic tenets of his treatment philosophy was patient self-government.

Like other individual programs that tend to change when a person responsible for them leaves the institution, Dr. Bierer's program underwent changes on his retirement in 1967. His successor, Dr. Felix Brown, tried to maintain a middle course between the extremes of over-permissiveness and regimentation. Patients of all kinds, including young neurotics, young people with character disorders, psychotic patients, and the aged, were all treated in one group, and all were encouraged to help one another. Large therapeutic groups were run on Monday, Tuesday, and Friday, each led by a different doctor. While the principles of each group were the same, the particular tone of the groups was influenced by whichever doctor was conducting the group. The doctors also conducted small therapeutic groups held every morning, during which free-wheeling discussions took place on a variety of subjects.

Dr. Brown also altered the practice of limiting overnight stays to occasional events under special circumstances. Instead, he set up a full-fledged inpatient unit, which housed eleven patients at the time of my first visit. The inpatient unit is comprised of a waiting room, three three-bed rooms, five single rooms, a waiting room which is also used as a sitting room, bathrooms, and a kitchen, which is used for preparing special diets as well as for cooking meals over the weekend when the main unit is closed. Some of the single rooms also double as doctor's offices. The doctor in charge over the weekend sleeps on the unit, and there are two trained staff members on duty at all times. Inpatients participate in the activities of the day hospital during the day. Some of the patients are actually night patients, who sleep on the inpatient unit at night and go to work during the day time. A few patients may be admitted for weekends only. The staff find the availability of the inpatient beds most useful for the brief hospitalization of patients experiencing an exacerbation of a psychosis or a deterioration of home circumstances.

At the time of my first visit, Marlborough Day Hospital was not actively engaged in research, but Brown indicated that the staff wished to establish an MRC unit for research in community psychiatry. In October 1969, he left Marlborough Day Hospital to become a consultant at the Royal Free Hospital. Since that time he has not been replaced, but Dr. Mayer, the child psychiatrist, has been acting senior consultant. The activities at Marlborough Day have since changed further, in that there are more small group meetings, more regular therapeutic community meetings, and more structure. In addition, the staff are trying to discontinue part-time attendance at the day hospital. The treatment unit, which was used for part-time hospitalization of some patients, is now regularly used as a full-fledged inpatient hospital where patients may occasionally stay up to as long as one year. Thus, the program, as it has progressed from Bierer to Brown to its current status, has moved from a kind of charismatic reflection of one man to a more highly organized and regulated activity, with less improvisation and spontaneity.

The future of the hospital is uncertain. Currently, the attitude of the Regional Hospital Board seems to be to end the tenure of the Marlborough Day Hospital as a free-standing, independent instutition. Rather, they wish to see it merge with a larger mental hospital or teaching hospital, whereby the facilities at Marlborough Day would become one aspect of the total program of the larger institution. They would also like the hospital to serve a specific catchment area. The Board may wish eventually to phase out Marlborough Day, because there are by now enough day hospitals affiliated with other institutions.

Among alternatives Marlborough Day has been exploring is an affiliation with the Tavistock Centre. They feel compatible with the latter institution, because their approaches are similar; that is, they emphasize psychotherapy rather than organic approaches. Since there are no inpatient or residential facilities at the Tavistock, an affiliation with Marlborough Day would supplement their program. In addition, the Tavistock sees Marlborough Day as a potential research unit. They would like to set up a family study unit in which whole families could be hospitalized, and the Marlborough staff agrees. The Regional Hospital Board, however, will make the final decision.

8

A program operated by the local authority*

NEWHAM BOROUGH

One of the most outstanding community-operated programs in England is found in Newham Borough, which is located in the east end of greater London. Newham was formed in 1965 by the joining of two neighboring county boroughs, East Ham (population 100,000) and West Ham (population 160,000), as part of a major reorganization of government in the London area (73). Both East Ham and West Ham were mainly working-class areas, although East Ham also included a middle-class element. Each borough had developed its own services prior to the amalgamation, but the community mental health service of West Ham was farther advanced than East Ham's. Thus the present service for Newham is really the West Ham scheme spread a little bit more thinly over the entire borough.

Much of the program is housed in a building acquired in December 1965 following the reorganization and known as the Newham Community Care Center. It is an old-fashioned building with bare steel girders across a large central hall, but it has acquired a welcoming appearance as the result of the decorating efforts of its occupants. It contains a number of small interviewing rooms, provides facilities for individual and group

*See also Chapter 13 for an in-depth study of community mental health services operated by a local authority (Camden Borough).

therapy as well as social group activities, and it serves as the home of the Young People's Counselling Service (YPCS). In this facility diagnostic assessments are carried out, multidisciplinary conferences are held, and meetings and group discussions with professional workers from the health department and other services are conducted. The center houses the community mental health staff, which consists of Dr. J. H. Kahn, the consultant psychiatrist in charge, a clinical psychologist, three educational psychologists, a child psychiatrist from the child guidance program, a child psychotherapist, and the various qualified and student psychiatric social workers.

When the Mental Health Act of 1959 imposed responsibilities upon the local authorities to develop community mental health programs, West Ham, with its long tradition of social experiment, enthusiastically took up the challenge. In planning the community mental health service, the MOH for West Ham at that time, Dr. F. Roy Dennison, used child guidance as a model. The child guidance approach is a multi-disciplinary system which views the child within a framework that encompasses family and school. Dr. Dennison felt that since the community mental-health approach views the adult's occupational life and family and social environment in a similar fashion, a multi-disciplinary framework was likewise called for. This approach would permit treatment to be directed to family interaction rather than to separate individuals, allow intervention at an earlier stage, and further the development of preventive services.

Since the implementation of the Seebohm Report in 1971, each local authority has been given the duty of creating a Social Service Department responsible for the rehabilitative social work and hostel services for the mentally ill and mentally handicapped. While in most local authorities a social worker has been appointed director, in Newham, Dennison has been made Director of the Social Service Department. The new Medical Officer of Health is Dr. Galbrey, formerly Deputy MOH under Dennison. Dennison's main interest has been and continues to be in mental health, while Galbrey is interested in working with the general practitioner. Galbrey has developed plans to create several health centers which would provide offices for the general practitioner and surround him with supporting services, including nursing personnel, and with consultative services by the various specialists. There are even plans for mobile child-guidance teams to visit the centers on a consultative basis.

As originally planned by Dennison, the community service had five aspects. First was to fulfil the statutory obligation for admission of the acutely ill patients to psychiatric hospitals and for the community care of patients discharged from the hospital but still unable to live independently in the community. At Newham plans for community care included provision of residential facilities, such as hostels for emotionally disturbed children, mentally handicapped children and adults, elderly patients with minor psychiatric disturbances, and patients with psychiatric illnesses not requiring hospital treatment at that particular time. Second were child-guidance clinics, operated along traditional lines, whose functions included casework with parents as well as treatment of children. Third were in-service training schemes for health visitors, assistant MOHs and professional workers in other departments of the local authority. Fourth were plans for consultation services for various kinds of local-authority staff such as health visitors, school medical officers, welfare officers, probation officers as well as volunteer workers, and organizations dealing with mental health programs. Finally, the service incorporated a previously existing coordinating committee made up of workers in different departments of the local authority and other voluntary bodies. The committee deals with multi-problem families with social, economic, and psychiatric problems.

At first, the psychiatric social workers manned a walk-in service for a growing number of patients presenting a variety of problems. Experienced in working with middle-class families, they anticipated difficulties with their new working-class clientele. But they found that many of the patients seeking help were atypical of the working class stereotype. The walk-ins included professional people and university students, as well as grammar school drop-outs entering employment. With those patients more characteristic of the working-class group, the expected problems did arise, particularly because of difficulties in communication, which led to inadequate definition of the client's problems. However, as the social workers' range of understanding increased, the clients became more individual and less examples of a stereotype, and communication could be established and needs identified.

In 1967 a Young Peoples Counselling Service was established, which young people were encouraged to approach directly rather than through an intermediary. The clientele of this service has generally tended to be young people starting to break away from families but not yet identified with an independent adult role. The majority of cases have been concerned with problems of interpersonal relationships.

Three local-authority social workers were attached to each of the three medical firms in the psychiatric hospital serving Newham, although there was no provision for joint appointments for social workers by the local authority and the hospital. Through their attendance at ward meetings and discharge conferences, the workers sought to establish links with the patients for whom they were responsible for aftercare, thus facilitating a continuity-of-care approach. In addition, nine maternal and child care clinics are spread out over the borough, and each has been assigned a particular social worker from the community mental health service.

The Newham community mental health service was from the first one of the few local authority programs to boast the services of a full-time psychiatrist, Dr. J. H. Kahn. The psychiatrist's function is purely consultative and administrative; he has no clinical responsibilities. I was informed that clinical responsibilities were the province of the psychiatrist on the staff of the mental hospitals, and that the community mental health program is a community agency where the responsibility for the "clients" belonged to the social worker. In this, the psychologist is in a rather ambiguous position, and one senses a great deal of friction between psychologists and social workers. At Newham, Dr. Kahn set up conjoint family-therapy groups in which a team of workers (psychiatrist, social worker, and psychologist) conduct joint-therapy interviews with whole families in selected cases.

Dr. Kahn came to the community mental health program with a background as medical director of a child guidance clinic, where he was accustomed to the role of leader of an interdisciplinary team whose diagnostic and therapeutic concepts were developed at weekly case conferences. In his community mental health post he has had to maintain contact also with the hospital psychiatric consultants who carry the clinical responsibility for all patients receiving inpatient or outpatient treatment. On the other hand, it is the psychiatric social worker who maintains contact with the family doctor and the family as a whole.

One of the most important functions of the community mental health service relates to liaison with mental hospitals. Traditionally, the statutory functions of emergency admission to mental hospitals and aftercare of discharged psychiatric patients were carried out by mental welfare officers (MWOs). In West Ham, Dr. Dennison felt that the function of the MWO in a community mental-health program could best be carried out by qualified psychiatric social workers (PSWs), and he therefore appointed psychiatric social workers to these positions. Initially, the main obstacle to this plan was the unavailability of qualified PSWs. People holding degrees or diplomas in social science were appointed to the posts and thereafter released on full salary for training courses which granted the mental health certificate in social work. Four such trainees were appointed in 1960, the first qualified worker returning to the service in 1962. This plan stimulated the recruitment of other newly qualified PSWs, and, as the staff grew in size, the easier recruiting became. At the time that Seebohm went into effect, Newham had the largest complement of *qualified* PSWs of any local authority in England. There was a complement of 25 workers, most of whom were fully qualified. The other disciplines were not nearly so well represented.

As a result of the psychiatric social-worker requirement, the MWO was no longer an officer who merely responds to a call for removal of a troublesome person in order to oblige the doctor or the patient's family. Rather, the PSWs brought a casework approach to the responsibilities of the MWO. They attempted to work with families in the hope of forestalling admissions, perhaps by helping the family to tolerate the patient through an acute stage of his illness. If hospitalization was necessary, they planned for the patient's admission and sought to prevent a division in the family or alienation of the patient. The caseworkers gradually extended their activities, as new areas of need were uncovered, in accordance with the special interests and abilities of the individual social workers.

This redefinition of the MWO role by the social workers was not always welcome, however. Because of the expectations of the community, based upon prior experience with the traditional MWO, the psychiatric social workers had to establish a new image of a service which dealt with calls on the basis of the long-term needs of the patient, his family, and the community, rather than merely in the context of providing the convenience of emergency admissions.

This adjustment worked out so well, however, that when the new Social Service Department was created as the result of the Seebohm Report (101), the duties of the MWO remained in the hands of the PSWs, despite the fact that in most other boroughs these duties were redistributed among the generic social workers, whatever their backgrounds.

Indeed, technically speaking, the expected redistribution of social-work duties following Seebohm has not occurred in Newham. This is largely due to Dr. Dennison, who has not pressed the "generic" concept. By allowing the workers to continue carrying out their former tasks, Dennison has avoided the "identity crisis" plaguing most of the new social service departments. There is, however, a continuing program of inservice education as well as an increased mingling of the social workers from diverse backgrounds. Dennison expects that this will result ultimately in a sharing of information about various fields of social work, thereby eventually permitting the generic concept to be put into practice.

In most local authorities the mental-health social workers have been at once the fewest in number and the most well trained. Long-standing rivalries have thus existed between them and their more numerous and less well-trained counterparts in the Welfare and Children's Departments. In most boroughs these rivalries sometimes resulted in open conflict, bitterness, and recrimination when the Social Service Department was created. Because of their greater numbers, the less trained workers from the Welfare and Children's Departments received most of the new administrative posts. In Newham, where PSWs are more numerous, the Mental Health Department contributed fully one-third of the 75 social workers to the new Social Service Department. This led to a more equitable distribution of administrative posts among the three groups and further reduced the stresses of reorganization.

The program at Newham has gone farther than any of the other centers I visited in developing a wide range of true community mental health services, emphasizing preventive and consultative services, and reaching almost every age group, with a genuine effort at continuity of care. Despite the upheavals of Seebohm, they have been able to maintain their leadership position as a community-operated mental health service.

Despite its rapid progress in many areas, Newham was slow to develop hostel accommodations for mentally disturbed and mentally handicapped individuals. This failure to carry out its statutory obligations and plans was due to indecision about the appropriate types of accommodations in which to invest. This situation was altered by a fortuitous circumstance. A series of slum clearance projects was undertaken in the borough, in which seven or eight new housing units were planned to be built on the cleared land over the next ten years. The housing authority requested consultation from the community mental health service about dealing with unruly tenants. As a consequence of this consultation activity, the housing authority agreed to provide hostels with 30 places in each of the housing units to be constructed. Authorization was also obtained for patients to live independently as individuals in these rental housing units. Facilities for 200 patients have already been completed; another hostel for 30 patients is in the process of being built, and two more are in the planning stages.

The hostel staff consists of the warden, deputy warden, domestic staff, and other supporting staff, as well as the visiting social workers responsible for the patients residing there. This staff is likewise responsible for liaison with the patients living in the independent housing units. The staff regularly provides consultation services to the housing authority on an ongoing basis and undertakes mental health efforts with the residents of the housing units such as arbitrating disputes between tenants.

The Newham program maintained an early active interest in the mentally retarded as well as the mentally ill. The mental health service was especially proud of its John F. Kennedy Center for mentally handicapped children. The Education Department, however, has now taken over responsibility for mentally retarded children. The new Social Service Department is responsible for providing facilities for mentally retarded adults. While these services are not as satisfactory as those for children, they have been greatly aided by the construction of the hostels mentioned above.

Probably because of Dr. Kahn's background, the community mental health service of Newham was one of the few which operated its own child guidance program. (Guidance clinics have been generally considered the province of the Education Department). Since psychiatric social workers and other guidance clinic staff members are assigned on a part-time basis, child guidance is brought into relation with the other elements of the community mental health service by the overlapping duties of the individual staff members. Indeed, educational psychologists, rarely found among the staffs of community mental health programs in England, play an active role in the Newham program because of its inclusion of child guidance.

Outreach projects for disturbed children, including those who get into trouble with the law, are increasing in number. A new psychiatric post has been created for a consultant to work with children either at the child guidance clinic, in the remand home, or in the borstal, which is a kind of prison for young offenders. The salary for the new post is derived from three sources: the Health Ministry for the prison work, the local authority for the work in the remand home, and the Regional Health Board for the child guidance clinic work. The support for the salaries of Dr. Kahn and Dr. Dennison comes entirely from the Regional Hospital Board.

9

Programs operated jointly by the mental hospital and the local authority

The statutory division of responsibility between the mental hospitals and the local authorities to provide community mental health services has impeded the development of integrated programs capable of providing continuity of care. It is therefore quite unusual to encounter true collaboration between mental-hospital and local-authority services, and the programs described are rather atypical. Each came about as the result of the determined efforts of an individual who could insure collaboration because he held an appointment with the local authority while serving as hospital superintendent.

NOTTINGHAM MENTAL HEALTH SERVICES

Nottingham comprises a hugh catchment area of 410,000 population, which includes both the city and the surrounding county. The region is densely populated, however, so that the actual geographic area covered is rather small. Indeed, the farthest distance between the mental hospital and the catchment area boundary is only nine miles.

The community mental health program was developed by Dr. Duncan MacMillan, who was Medical Superintendent of the Mapperley Hospital and also held the post of Mental Health Officer of the local authority. Dr. MacMillan was able to retain the cooperation of the manage-

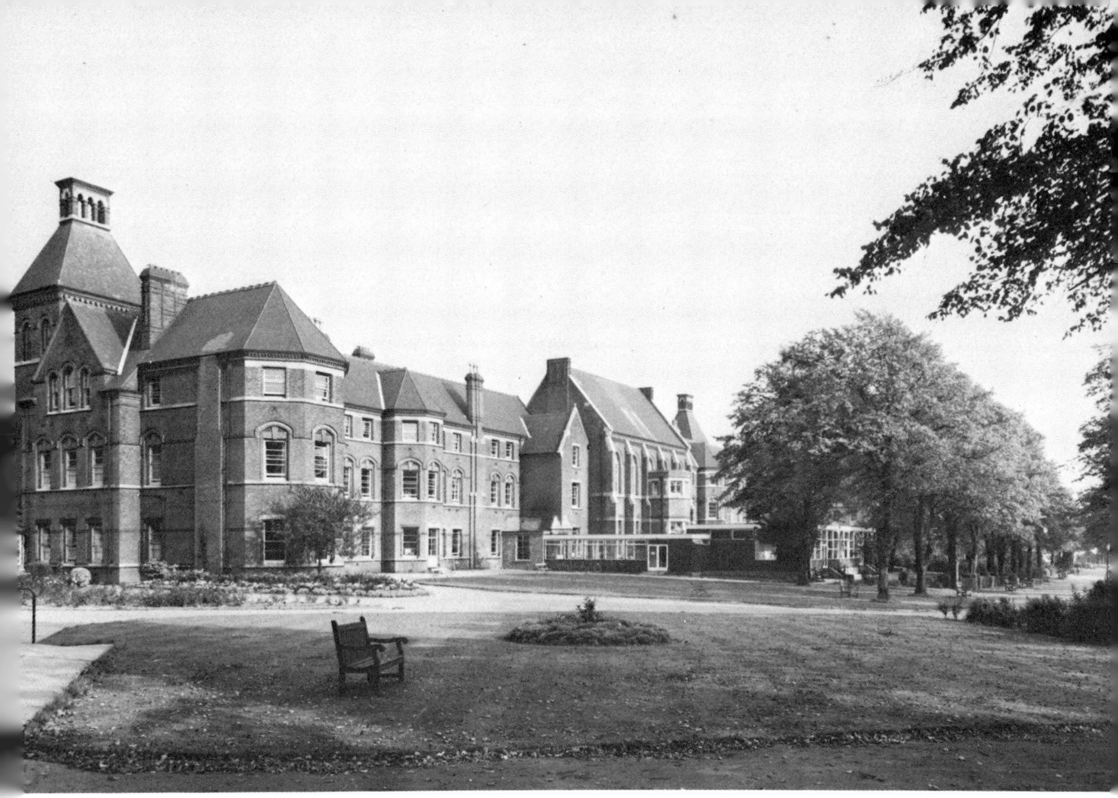

Mapperley Hospital, Nottingham. (*Courtesy of Maurice Baird, M.D.*)

ment committee of Mapperley Hospital after the position of Medical Superintendent was abolished; although there was a period of friction with a traditional Medical Officer of Health, this situation improved significantly when the incumbent was replaced by a younger man. A good relationship was subsequently maintained between the hospital and the local authority. The local authority staff attended meetings at the hospital every two or three weeks, and the social workers of the hospital and those of the local authority got along very well together. This fortunate state of affairs was able to survive the departure of MacMillan. Dr. G. Maurice Baird, the senior consultant at Mapperley Hospital at the time of my 1969 visit, carried on the efforts to maintain a comprehensive jointly operated service (though the major leadership role was clearly centered in the hospital).

Twenty years ago Mapperley had 1,300 beds. This number was steadily reduced, so that at the time of my visit only 650 beds were in use. However, the hospital maintained responsibility for a tremendous number of outpatients and day patients. It is located very near the center of the city within pleasant grounds. In addition to the usual traditional impatient facilities, the hospital maintains a specialized addiction unit, a children's unit, an adolescent unit, a neurosis unit, and a male and a female day center. Among the most unusual facets of the Mapperley program are the three geriatric day centers.

The hospital has ten consultant psychiatrists, seven registrars, and four visiting general practitioners. Three of the consultants are on 9/11 time. The clinical services are organized into three firms, each with three consultants. One consultant is on emergency call each day to the Health Department. The hospital employs four social workers who were assigned full time to the local-authority mental health section. There are also two student social workers, one of whom is assigned to the children's and adolescent units. There is a "Department of Resettlement," which is really a community nursing program whose task it is to resettle long-stay patients in the community. This service is under the leadership of a chief nurse, who has one deputy and two part-time nurses. Patients are placed with landlords and landladies in the community. Most of the patients receive treatment on a day basis at the hospital's Industrial Therapy Unit but reside in the community lodgings. The community nurses visit the patients in their lodgings, counsel them, administer medication, and try to settle any problems with the landlords. If the landlords become too upset by the patients or if they go on holiday, the patients are returned to the hospital temporarily.

A weekly case conference is held at which all available staff are present. Each firm in turn presents a case which is discussed by the entire group.

The special addiction unit was set up to handle alcoholics and drug addicts residing in the southern half of the Sheffield region, but because of the paucity of such facilities, the unit actually accepts patients from a much larger area. The children's unit accepts small numbers of children up to age twelve who are considered likely to benefit from inpatient treatment. Diagnostic categories include autistic children as well as behavior disorders. The adolescent unit takes children between the ages of twelve and fifteen. There are no facilities for looking after adolescents who become physically ill, however, and they must be sent to adult wards for treatment.

There are seldom more than one or two involuntary patients in the hospital, and all doors are unlocked. There are no seclusion rooms, all of which have been converted to other purposes. Available treatment includes electroshock, drugs, occupational therapy, and some psychotherapy, chiefly in groups. The major therapeutic emphasis, however, is undoubtedly vested in the industrial therapy program.

Day Unit for Industrial Therapy

The industrial therapy program is based in a special "day unit for industrial therapy" (DUIT), which is run very much on the lines of a factory. Patients clock in and out, are paid on a piecework basis, and earn from 25 new pence to £2.00 weekly. Even the dining unit is operated therapeutically, as a patient-staffed canteen. There are 109 day patients and approximately 50 inpatients working in the DUIT. There are 10 staff under the overall direction of the industrial manager, who began as a male psychiatric nurse, then went into occupational therapy, and finally became interested in industrial therapy.

There is a regular flow of work at the unit, and sometimes it is even necessary to turn down some requests. Activities include packing ladies' underwear, carding pencils, putting polyethylene bags onto wickets, packaging eyebrow pencils, assembling pens, packing material for export, etc. The patients also repair furniture for the hospital and do finishing work on projects made at the Blind Institute. Patients make novelty items sold aboard the Cunard Line ships, packing, pricing, and completely finishing the product. They operate a complete print shop, in which all of the hospital's printing is done, and a shoe repair shop, but these latter activities are classified as occupational therapy rather than industrial therapy, so that the patients working there will not be called out on strike in the event of a union dispute.*

The Disablement Resettlement Officer visits the unit every week to learn who is fit and ready for a job; he then tries to find appropriate employment. In the first year of operation of the Industrial Therapy Unit, 75 patients were placed on jobs in the community, and very few of these have returned to the hospital. The caliber of patient being discharged has declined, however, so that currently a much larger proportion of those placed in jobs return to the hospital. This seems to be the consequence of having creamed off the healthiest patients during the first year and getting closer to the bottom of the chronicity barrel with each successive year. Most of the day patients live in hostels in the community, and the unit is currently negotiating for a community-based sheltered workshop in the hope of reducing the rate of return.

Geriatric Program

Unlike most of the mental hospitals in England, the Mapperley staff do not regard geriatric problems as inappropriate for a mental hospi-

*The industrial therapy program has the blessing of the unions, but the workers are naturally concerned about competition from low-paid patient labor. Hence, in the event of a strike in a particular field, industrial therapy programs in similar fields are closed down.

tal, and the psychiatrists work closely with the geriatricians. Mapperley, in fact, has developed a highly elaborate program. There is a day geriatric ward accommodating 60-70 patients, and operating 24 hours a day, seven days per week. It is used by people living alone, including senile patients. Patients are collected at their lodgings in the morning and returned there by ambulance. The hours of operation permit full flexibility, enabling each patient to attend the program for as few or as many hours per day as are required, even up to complete 24-hour hospitalization. For the most part, however, there are two programs, a "short day" beginning at 9:00 A.M. and extending to 3:30 or 4:30 in the afternoon, during which patients receive morning refreshments, lunch, and afternoon tea; and a "long day" beginning at 7:30 A.M. and extending to 7:30 or 8:00 P.M., during which patients receive, in addition, breakfast and supper. Eight side rooms in the day unit provide sleeping accommodations, enabling the unit to accept 24-hour patients for limited periods. These rooms may be used for keeping patients for a few weeks at a time, in order to give families a vacation from the patient who otherwise lives with them. They are also used to provide a cooling-off period for a family who may have become intolerant of the patient, or to re-stabilize a patient who has begun to decompensate. If patients become physically ill, they are transferred to the sick ward.

Three nurses, two cadets, and one ward maid staff the geriatric day center. A social worker is also attached to the ward. The day unit is fully staffed during the day and afternoon, and there is a night nurse on duty. All kinds of cases are accepted. Most of the patients live alone. When they arrive in the morning, the patients are given a wash and brushup followed by morning coffee. A variety of activities includes raffles, hymn singing, outings, and occupational therapy. Patients participate in these activities according to their ability. Some sit and read or knit, others watch television, while a few merely nap in their chairs.

The hospital provides outpatient services within the community. These include diagnostic and consultative services as well as aftercare programs for discharged patients.

Community volunteers also take part in the mental health program. The Nottingham "League of Friends" supplies to patients special amenities not obtainable from ordinary benefits, arranges visits to inpatients, and facilitates mental health education. It has raised funds to build a cafeteria and gift shop on the hospital grounds.

The local authority provides ambulances to bring the patients to and from the hospital; the hospital pays all other costs. Nuffield House is another geriatric day center which operates along similar lines, but this unit makes a fixed charge of approximately five new pence per day per patient. There is more intensive emphasis on occupational therapy at Nuffield House, whose patients tend to be better preserved.

Effects of the Seebohm Report

Prior to the changes brought about by the Seebohm Report (101), the Local Authority Mental Health Department had the primary obligation for arranging admission to the hospital. The traditional MWO was responsible both for seeing that the mentally retarded were properly cared for and for expediting admission of the mentally ill to mental hospitals. He also had certain responsibilities for their aftercare. In Nottingham, the MWO was more active in aftercare than in most other places in England. While the MWO's duties were not assigned to social workers by the local authority, hospital social workers were assigned to the local authority staffs to perform psychiatric social work functions. A close liaison was maintained between the hospital and the Local Authority Mental Health Department, which functioned almost as if it were a division of the hospital. Notes regarding admission or discharge of patients were exchanged between the local authority and the hospital to keep both organizations informed as to the patient's status.

The Local Authority Mental Health Section, now a part of the new Social Service Department, still has close links with the hospital, but the relationship is not as good as formerly for several reasons. First, although the Social Service Department is now organized into six subcatchment areas, the hospital has not reorganized its services to correspond with them.

The hospital is currently organized into specialized wards, such as the addiction ward, the geriatric ward, and the adolescent ward, each of which provides specialized services for particular groups of patients in a centralized fashion. It would not be feasible to decentralize these services in order to organize the hospital along unit lines corresponding to the subcatchment areas of the new Social Service Department. If each specialized service were to be represented in each unit, fragmentation and deterioration of service would result. The relationship between the hospital and local authority has therefore become more difficult. The lack of correspondence between the areas of responsibility of the local-authority social workers and the pattern of organization of the hospital has led to confusion and some friction. The hospital must now deal with two separate social service departments, one for the city of Nottingham, and one for the county. In addition, the newly augmented staffs of these social service departments are more interested in expanding their relationships with the general practitioners than in strengthening their ties to the hospital, despite the fact that the directors of both social service departments are members of the Hospital Management Committee.

The hospital social workers have also become upset since the implementation of Seebohm. Many feel threatened by the changes. The local-authority social service departments pay a higher salary scale than does the hospital, and many social workers are attracted by this economic incentive but are nevertheless unable to come to a decision to move into the community. They are reluctant to relinquish their identity, area of interest, and expertise as psychiatric social workers in favor of becoming generic social workers. In addition, they prefer clinical work with patients to the administrative responsibilities often assigned to workers with considerable experience. For the time being, the hospital social workers have elected to remain but are unhappy that it requires a financial sacrifice to do so.

In consequence of Seebohm (101), the responsibilities of the MOH have been sharply reduced, as has been his budget. He is now called "Community Physician," but his duties are not well defined and there is a possibility that, with the anticipated reorganization of the health service, the post may be eliminated altogether. As matters currently stand, medical care in the community is becoming increasingly concentrated in health centers staffed by general practitioners, as primary physicians, whose services are augmented by those of the social workers and health visitors. Despite the general practitioners' interest in emphasizing this aspect of their responsibilities, the social service departments have not had adequate numbers of social workers to assign. Fortunately, the health visitors have a strong psychiatric orientation.

In addition to changes in the hospital-community relationship resulting from the Seebohm Report (101), other organizational changes have recently occurred. According to Dr. G. Maurice Baird, a huge new Hospital Management Committee, known as the Trent Vale Hospital Group, has assumed responsibility for six hospitals including Mapperley, Saxondale, the Coppice Hospital, St. Francis Hospital, Balderton Hospital, and Aston Hall Hospital. The last two are hospitals for the mentally subnormal. Saxondale is a mental hospital serving the outlying county beyond Mapperley's catchment area. Mapperley and Saxondale have been linked together as a temporary measure to provide jointly the psychiatric services ultimately to be provided by a new 150-bed psychiatric unit to be constructed at the Nottingham General Hospital. The plan is for the medical services in the area to be concentrated at three general hospitals: Nottingham General, which is to be the district general hospital; the Nottingham City Hospital; and a new 1,500-bed teaching hospital for the medical school of Nottingham University.

Pending completion of this teaching hospital, 120 beds have been set aside on the south side of Mapperley for the use of the students and medical school. This has necessitated a considerable expenditure for conference rooms, students' rooms, etc. The medical school, which opened in 1970, has placed more emphasis on psychiatry than most medical schools in Britain generally do. Community medicine and psychiatry are introduced during the preclinical years. The new professor, Dr. J. E. Cooper, is already in residence, has a house on the hospital grounds, and is working at Mapperley. There will be approximately 150 students enrolled per year in the new medical school.

The plan to concentrate inpatient psychiatric beds at the district general hospital and at the new medical school has created significant anxiety among the staff psychiatrists at Mapperley because of the prospect that their posts will be phased out of existence. However, certain developments have been somewhat reassuring to them. The projected number of psychiatric beds was originally developed as part of the Hospital Building Programme of 1966 (52), but there has been such a marked increase in population that it is likely that more psychiatric beds will be required than was at first anticipated. Further, there has been a significant delay in the construction of the 150-bed unit at Nottingham General Hospital chiefly due to financial problems. The annual budget of the Health Ministry (around £2 billion) is not likely to increase, despite the new construction resulting from the Ministry's efforts to develop regional and district hospitals. Consequently, the closure of Mapperley and Saxondale hospitals, in favor of the district general-hospital psychiatric unit, will undoubtedly be delayed longer than had been originally forecast. Even should the closure occur sooner than is now expected, it is likely that the personnel currently at Mapperley will constitute the staff for the new district general-hospital psychiatric unit. Another reassuring development is that many Mapperley consultants have been offered teaching assignments with the medical students, and a number of the psychiatrists are consequently hopeful of receiving faculty appointments with the new medical school.

Other prospective changes also have created an air of uncertainty. The implementation of the Redcliffe-Maud (58) proposal for government reorganization will combine the city and county services into one large region, further complicating the relationships between the hospital and the community. It will mean that the two social service departments will be merged into one, and there undoubtedly will be an upheaval among the social workers. Nevertheless, the already existing Mapperley-Saxondale relationship would fit easily into the reorganization pattern, and it would be easier to relate to a single social service department than to the present two. Currently, each hospital is in somewhat of a quandary as to how to relate to the two social service departments and have not had any guidance along these lines from the Health Ministry.

The budgetary problems, however, make it more difficult to obtain funds to maintain the old structures which frequently require repair and renovation. Thus, it is likely that both Mapperley and Saxondale Hospitals will eventually be phased out of existence, although some have estimated it will be fifteen years before this actually occurs.

CROYDON MENTAL HEALTH SERVICES

The most outstanding example of cooperation between mental hospitals and local authority services is found in the London borough of Croydon. It came about through the pioneering efforts of Dr. Anthony R. May, who is responsible for promoting many of the ideas later widely adopted in community mental health programs. Dr. May was in a peculiarly fortunate position to institute these innovations, since he served as superintendent of the mental hospital, psychiatric advisor to the National Hospital Board, and psychiatric director for the Local Authority Health Services. May viewed the mental hospital as merely a part of the total community mental-health treatment program. Indeed, he considered it undesirable for the mental hospital to dominate the pattern, believing that the hospital doctors tended to be more concerned with the institution than the community. He also objected to outpatient services as hospital extensions, and was critical of day hospitals operated like chronic mental hospital wards. He felt such programs should be community facilities operated as part of a community mental health center. May considered rehabilitation to be the province of the social worker, with the psychiatrist being most active during the acute clinical phases of psychiatric illness. He advocated home visits by nurses. He considered that the psychiatrist should be the leader of a treatment team coordinating the efforts of the various members. He proposed that several treatment teams, functioning as units, serve geographic segments of the community population (the catchment area concept) and that there be a corresponding unit system of bed distribution at the mental hospital as well.

Although May is no longer at Croydon (he was promoted to the Ministry of Health and subsequently moved on to the World Health Organization), most of his ideas have come to full fruition. Since 1959, a close integration between services of the Warlingham Park Hospital and the local authority mental health services has developed into an extensive network of community facilities. This close cooperation is exemplified in the excellent working relationship between Dr. S. L. Wright, the Medical Officer of Health for Croydon, and Dr. J. D. W. Fisher, consultant psychiatrist of the hospital, who serves as psychiatric advisor to the borough; the relationship is represented symbolically by Rees House.

Warlingham Park Hospital

Croydon's population of approximately 330,000 is served by Warlingham Park Hospital, an 850-bed institution, which admits approximately 1,000 patients per year. Even before Dr. May, Warlingham Park was a pioneer hospital under Dr. T. P. Rees (for whom Rees House is named), who was at the forefront of the open-hospital movement. Indeed, there have been no closed wards at Warlingham Park since 1954. Currently, Warlingham Park is organized on the basis of five clinical firms, each headed by a consultant psychiatrist. Each consultant has an intake day and assumes general treatment responsibilities for all admissions on that day (unless the patient is admitted after a domiciliary visit, in which case the consultant who made the visit retains responsibility for that patient). There is no organization along geographic unit lines as envisioned by May; this is one of the rare instances where his plan has not been put into practice. There are special functional units at the hospital for alcoholic and geriatric patients, as well as a rehabilitation unit. In addition to his general responsibilities for the patients assigned to his clinical firm, each consultant has a special responsibility such as community work, the alcoholic unit, psychogeriatrics, or the day hospital.

Warlingham Park operates graded workshops for industrial therapy, as well as traditional occupational therapy and art therapy programs. As patients show improvement in their industrial therapy assignments, they are promoted to higher grades. When they reach the highest grade they are transferred to an assessment and rehabilitation center in the community, where again they are assigned to workshops on a graded basis. When they reach the top rung, the patients are sent out into open employment or sheltered workshops in the community.

At the time of my first visit, there were 33 social workers employed jointly by Warlingham Park and the local authority, of whom 15 were qualified psychiatric social workers and 6 were mental welfare officers. Since the implementation of the Seebohm Report in 1971, the Children's Department, Welfare Department, and the Mental Health Section of the Health Department have been combined to form the Department of Social Services. There are now approximately 100 social workers of various grades including former MWOs, psychiatric social workers, and students, and all of the workers hold joint appointments with Warlingham Park Hospital and the local authority. The social workers are assigned to clinical teams in varying numbers according to the number of patients for which the team is responsible. In addition, each social work team is assigned community aftercare responsibility for a geographical segment of Croydon Borough (catchment areas). There is a social-work intake team, whose job it is to screen patients referred by non-medical sources, such as the Probation Department, the Social Service Department, voluntary agencies, neighbors, employers, relatives, etc. Since the patients for whom each team is responsible are being treated in various hospitals or community facilities, each unit decides for itself how its work assignments are to be divided. Weekly consultation sessions are held for the social workers by

Dr. Fisher in his capacity as psychiatric advisor to the borough. The workers maintain a case load of about 1,400 patients, of whom 500 are mentally subnormal. There are approximately 1,100 new referrals per year.

In addition to Warlingham Park, hospital facilities include a twelve-bed general hospital ward in Croydon at Mayday Hospital, for female short-stay patients (average length of stay is four weeks). There are approximately 150 admissions a year to Mayday Hospital. A thirty-bed psychogeriatric assessment unit has been opened at Queens Hospital, a geriatric institution.

Rees House

The main day-hospital, operated by Warlingham Park, is located in the new mental health center at Rees House, which also contains the headquarters for the local authority services. (The original day-hospital, "The Oaks," opened in 1955, moved to larger quarters in 1961, and finally to Rees House in 1968.) While the hospital and local authority services are each located in different parts of the building, there is ready access from one part to another and free, active communication and collaboration between the staffs of each.

The facilities include an occupational therapy room, which contains facilities for light industrial therapy work, such as a printing press, a sewing machine, and a kitchen for cooking classes. There is also a large room where group therapy sessions are held daily between 9:30 and 10:30 A.M. Often these sessions are conducted as therapeutic community conferences, with various staff members being present to discuss problems with the patients. This room is also used for physical exercise and general relaxation. A canteen on the first floor is used by patients and staff alike. Also on the first floor are two smaller group rooms. The second floor consists mainly of psychologists' offices and interviewing rooms.

About fifty day places are provided both for the treatment of acute problems and rehabilitation of the chronically ill. There are approximately 200 admissions to the day hospital program per year. The program is organized along therapeutic community lines and conducted by a multidisciplinary team of social workers, nurses, psychologists, and psychiatric registrars. Dr. Fisher is the only psychiatric consultant. In addition, the day hospital makes use of an extensive outpatient nursing program, wherein psychiatric nurses visit patients in their homes, make evaluations, and administer medication. Nurses also make home visits to follow up patients who fail to attend their scheduled day hospital sessions. Therapeutic social clubs, clinics, and ambulatory group therapy programs are also conducted at the day hospital, as well as a play group for the children of adult patients.

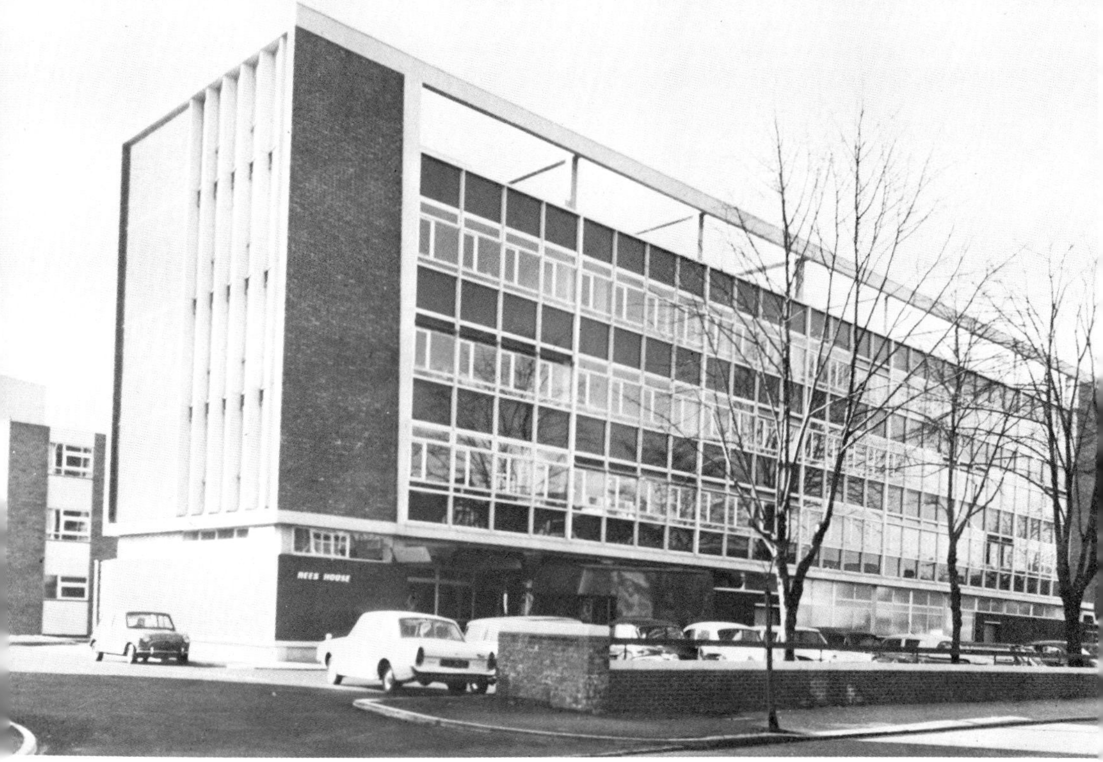

Rees House, Croydon. (*Courtesy of J.D.W. Fisher, M.D.*)

While electroshock treatment is rarely used, there is extensive utilization of Modecate, a long-acting phenothiazine administered by injection. Although he has not conducted a controlled study, Fisher has changed his attitude from one of skepticism to a positive endorsement of this medication which he believes to be a major factor in permitting a large number of patients to remain in the community.

Although there are electroconvulsive therapy (ECT) facilities at Rees House, this form of treatment is rarely administered there. When ECT is needed on an outpatient basis, it is usually done at the Croydon General Hospital about a mile away. Patients come for various amounts of time, some five days per week, some three days, and others for shorter periods. A few of the patients reside at Warlingham Park, using the institution more or less as a hostel, obtaining their treatment at the day hospital. Most patients make their own way to Rees House, although some are brought by ambulance. Patients arrive at 9:00 A.M. and leave at 4:00 P.M. A five-day emergency service is open until 9:00 P.M. Evening activities at the center include social clubs and groups run by the social workers. On Tuesday evening there is a special group for alcoholics. Staffing includes one part-time and three full-time psychiatric nurses, two occupational therapists assisted by a student occupational therapist, two specially assigned psychiatric social workers and other social workers from Warlingham Park on a part-time basis, two part-time psychiatric registrars, and the consultant, Dr. Fisher.

At Warlingham Park Hospital Fisher conducts a consultation service for the social work firms and makes domiciliary visits in doubtful cases. Whereas the other consultants deal mainly with the social workers assigned to their own clinical firms, Fisher consults with all of the social workers assigned to the various catchment areas because of his community responsibility. He sees about 200 domiciliary cases per year for evaluation. About one-third of these are admitted to Warlingham Park; the others are assigned to be followed by the social workers, admitted directly for treatment in day hospitals, or assigned to the clinics or other facilities.

Fisher gives 9/11 time to the National Health Service, in addition to which he sees about six private patients per week (mostly for psychotherapy). He goes into Warlingham Park each day but does not have much direct contact with patients there, other than those he admits on that day. Fisher conducts a clinic on Monday afternoon, when he sees one or two new referrals for evaluation as well as other patients for psychotherapy, drug treatment, etc. He conducts a weekly clinic in the general hospital as well. He also attends a Friday morning group meeting at the day hospital and another day-hospital staff meeting, which the entire team attends. In addition, he is in communication with general practictioners who request domiciliary visits.

I attended one of the weekly staff meetings at Rees House at which admission of new patients to the day hospital was discussed. The meeting was conducted by Fisher and was attended by a senior registrar; a registrar; the Disablement Resettlement Officer; three psychiatric social workers, another social worker, and a social work student; the nursing sister in charge of the day hospital, plus another nurse; a psychologist; a senior occupational therapist; and an occupational therapy student. Another psychiatric social worker, who was soon to begin employment at Rees House, also attended the conference as a visitor. The registrar and senior registrar spend part of their time at Warlingham Park Hospital and part at Rees House.

During the meeting a brief discussion was held on each new admission or readmission. The staff maintains a bulletin board with a rather complex system of notations, using different colored plastic cards, for keeping track of the day patients according to days of attendance and staff members responsible for the patient.

The staff meeting was followed by a case conference, attended by Fisher, the senior registrar, and the nurses who are engaged in making home visits as part of the aftercare program. During the meeting, one of the nurses discussed her entire caseload, asking advice from the doctors regarding problems she had come across or making appointments for the patients to see the doctor if this was felt necessary. Each week a different nurse reviews her caseload with the other nurses and the doctors. Nurses are usually assigned to the aftercare program on a rotation basis, spending three months doing home visits and the rest of the time on duty at Warlingham Park. The nurses say that they enjoy the home visit assignments and appeared to be quite conscientious in carrying out their responsibilities. They do not object to the large amount of travelling involved in making the visits and seem to believe they are making an important contribution to the maintenance of the patients in the community.

Other Day Hospitals and Services

In addition to the main day hospital at Rees House, there are three smaller day hospitals. The Crescent Day Hospital/Center accommodates 40 patients and serves a rapidly expanding new housing estate in New Addington. The Purley House was opened in October 1969, accommodates 50 patients, and serves the southern part of the borough. In 1970, the Oaks was reopened as a 50-place day hospital which serves the remaining area of Croydon. The Crescent and Purley are under the management of one consultant team, and the other two day hospitals are shared equally by a pair of consultant teams.

About 30 outpatient clinic sessions are conducted each week, with approximately 15,000 visits per year. There are around 1,000 new patient referrals annually to these clinics, which are based at Mayday Hospital and the other day hospitals. These clinics are in addition to the previously mentioned emergency clinic based at the day hospital.

There is also a child guidance clinic which sees approximately 300 new referrals each year. This clinic is based at the Warlingham Park Hospital but is closely linked with the local authority. It is jointly financed by the Education Department, which supplies the psychologists, and the Warlingham Park Hospital. The clinic maintains a day center for children and conducts groups for joint treatment of mothers and children.

The outpatient psychiatric nursing service established in 1954 was the first of its kind. Four full-time experienced psychiatric nurses provide aftercare in the community for some 300 patients. This approach has been found particularly valuable for supervising medication and for detecting early relapses in chronic patients. The visits are made unannounced rather than by appointment; they take place weekly, fortnightly, monthly, or bi-monthly, and the length of each visit varies between 10 and 30 minutes.

Social Service Department: Organization

As previously noted, the local authority services are based at Rees House, which is jointly financed by Warlingham Park Hospital and the local authority. When the Seebohm Report went into effect, the Welfare Department, Children's Department, and the Mental Health Section of the Health Department were combined into the Social Service Department. The new director of Social Services is Mr. G. H. Borroff. Each of the four main divisions of the department is under an assistant director.

Field Work and Domiciliary Services

Following the recommendations of Seebohm, this division will establish four area offices adjacent to or near the existing day centers, and their boundaries will be contiguous with the five subcatchment areas of the hospital. Each office will have one or two teams of social workers according to the size of the area, and the total number of social workers will vary, from 14 in one area to 24 in each of the other three areas.

Residential and Specialist Care Services

The local authority operates three basic types of residential programs: boarding-out, group homes, and hostels. The boarding-out scheme, inaugurated in 1962, provides accommodations for about 75 patients, of whom approximately 40% are mentally subnormal. The patients are boarded out with one of approximately 40 officially accredited landladies. The program is subsidized by the local authority, which employs two boarding-out officers to recruit and support landladies and to place the patients. Over one half of the placements in the boarding-out scheme are long term.

There are 5 small group homes, which are ordinary houses owned by the local authority, some of which are supervised and some unsupervised. Each provides accommodation for 6 to 8 patients. Additionally, the local authority maintains 20 places in a leased hostel operated by the Mental After-Care Association and 7 places in a hostel for alcoholics operated by the Richmond Fellowship. Both hostels are located in Croydon Borough. There is a hospital for senile and psychogeriatric patients next to Rees House, which is visited by the psychiatrist every week. A new home for the aged mentally infirm was opened in 1968, which provides 39 places, and a hostel for 12 working male patients was opened in 1970, in spite of some difficulty with the local residents.

Day Care Services for the Handicapped

This division is concerned mainly with training and rehabilitating the mentally and physically handicapped. In addition to Rees House and other day centers already mentioned, Croydon has a complex network of facilities for all aspects of industrial rehabilitation and training supported by the Department of Employment. The local authority operates the Unified Industrial Work Service consisting of the Crosfield Industrial Unit, the Waylands Craftwork Training and Social Center, and the Cherry Orchard Advanced Adult Training Center. The Crosfield Unit, established in 1962, has gradually expanded to serve as the administrative headquarters and coordinating agency for all contract work undertaken in these centers. It is headed by an Assistant Director of Social Services, who holds a joint appointment with the local authority and the hospital.

In one section of the Crosfield Industrial Unit, there is a sheltered workshop providing 110 places for severely disabled persons. Forty percent of the patients are mentally ill, another 40% are subnormals, and 20% are physically handicapped. Fares to and from the factory are reimbursed, and midday meals are supplied free of charge. Most employees live in their own homes or hostels, although a small group who are awaiting hostel places attend directly from the local psychiatric hospital.

Another section, called the Assessment and Rehabilitation Unit, accommodates about 20 rehabilitees. Realistic working conditions are simulated, productivity is measured, and the reaction of workers to stress and industrial pressure is evaluated. They are responsible for their own transportation to and from the unit. Some attend from their own homes, while others come directly from the hospital. The disablement resettlement officer attached to the unit helps to place them in jobs when they are ready for discharge.

The Waylands Craftwork Training and Social Center is a unique, purpose-built facility opened in 1967. It has two wings, one for 85 physically handicapped persons and one for 120 mentally subnormal individuals. There are joint social facilities. Trainees attend from their own homes and are conveyed to and from the center by special coaches. Those capable of making their own way are encouraged to do so and are reimbursed. The program emphasizes work and socio-educational subjects. A resident warden and social organizer are employed to develop leisure and recreational activities for disabled Croydon residents. Evening and weekend clubs provide entertainment.

The Cherry Orchard Advanced Adult Training Center provides work-oriented training for up to 100 mentally handicapped adults and functions as an intermediate center between the Waylands and Crosfield. Many trainees make their own way to and from the center, although busses are provided for those unable to do so. (Weekly merit payments range from £1.25 to £2.00).

A psychogeriatric day center was opened in 1968, which provides 50 places. It is administered by the local authority, but the hospital sends nursing and medical staff. Approximately 25% of the hospital admissions are over 65 years of age. This day center and a newly opened psychogeriatric assessment unit are expected to reduce the number of elderly patients at Warlingham Park.

Finance and Administration

This division of the Social Service Department is responsible for the budgetary control of a gross expenditure of £2 million per year and staff administration, involving over 1,000 people.

According to Fisher, voluntary services in Croydon were originally set up as a two-year pilot project sponsored by the National Association of Mental Health and subsidized by the King Edward Fund. Because of its success, the Croydon Volunteer Aid Project was placed on a permanent basis in April 1970. A full-time coordinator is employed jointly by the hospital and local authority to recruit, train, and supervise the volunteer workers in the mental health field, and to supplement statutory services both in the hospital and community setting. Over 900 volunteers have been recruited and about 47 organizations have become involved. There are flourishing branches of the Samaritans, Alcoholics Anonymous, Gamblers Anonymous, the Society for Mentally Handicapped Children, etc., in Croydon. There are also close, but informal, links between the voluntary societies and the Crosfield Industrial Unit.

The borough maintains periodic publicity campaigns designed to educate the community to the services offered. Particularly, they seek to obtain referrals from general practitioners and others in the community before the patients reach a crisis. General practitioners vary in their interest in psychiatric problems. For example, all of the Croydon general practitioners (around 300), were invited to a barbecue, but only 30-35 attended. A study has been initiated to evaluate referrals made by general practitioners. There is an effort to educate the general practitioner to refer cases to the social workers rather than to the psychiatrists, but some general practitioners will deal only with doctors. Nevertheless, the social workers maintain an extensive telephone liaison with the general practitioners, and Dr. Fisher conducts an active domiciliary consultation service with them.

10

General hospital programs

Probably the most extensive utilization of general hospital psychiatric facilities is found in the Manchester region (28, 103). As early as 1948 the Manchester Regional Hospital Board decided against preserving the system of large, remote mental hospitals and moved instead to develop psychiatric units at the local general hospitals. Their objective was to reintegrate psychiatry with the rest of medicine and also to develop a close working relationship between psychiatry and the public health and welfare services operated by the borough councils.

Before the advent of the National Health Service, each community in the Manchester region, as elsewhere in Britain, tended to have two general hospitals. One was usually a voluntary hospital, and the second was a public hospital containing a poor-law section for treatment of the indigent chronically ill, including mentally ill and mentally subnormal patients. These poor-law units also traditionally cared for the homeless and those requiring long-term custodial care. The units were abolished by the Manchester Regional Hospital Board, and the buildings housing them were converted into psychiatric units for the adjacent general hospitals. Although the units are not located within the general hospital proper, they are on the same campus so that communication between the staffs is not too difficult.

The Manchester region comprises a population of some four-and-one-half million, including the city of Manchester with a population of 700,000. The region is highly urban and industrial and densely populated. It is divided into a number of political subdivisions under borough councils which are responsible for providing community services. The hospitals are governed by local hospital management committees responsible to the Manchester Regional Hospital Board. Several general hospitals are linked together in administrative groupings, and at least one hospital in each group has a psychiatric unit which serves a defined catchment area population of 150,000 to 350,000.

The goal of the National Health Service to reduce the ratio of psychiatric beds to 1.8 per thousand of population (50, 106) will be far surpassed by the Manchester region, which expects to require only 0.5 beds per thousand (this does not take into account the backlog of chronic patients left over from former years, however).

Two community mental health programs in the Manchester region utilizing general hospital psychiatric facilities will be described: the program at Blackburn and the one at Salford. While both programs are regarded as outstanding, they are nevertheless characteristic of the general approach of the various communities of the region. Finally, an unusual and pace-setting program in London will be described.

BLACKBURN

Several large general hospitals serve the Blackburn area. The Queen's Park Hospital with 600 beds is the only one with a psychiatric unit. The psychiatric program serves a catchment area population of 250,000 with only 107 beds and has completely obviated the need for a separate mental hospital. In addition to the inpatient service there is a day treatment program, an Alcoholics Anonymous program together with a social club for the spouses of alcoholics, and also another therapeutic social club. In addition, there is an outpatient clinic for diagnostic evaluations, followup, and aftercare. Most of the treatment offered in the clinic consists of group psychotherapy plus a great deal of drug management and much outpatient electroshock therapy. About 500 new patients per year are admitted to the outpatient services, and 40-60 patients are seen each day. In addition, the local authority operates several hostels in the community as lodgings for mental patients.

Of the 107 inpatient beds, 40% are occupied by long-stay, chronically ill patients. However, the actual time of residence on the inpatient unit for these patients is usually less than twelve months, because most of the chronic patients are referred to the day treatment program, where they then continue to be carried for many years. Some of these chronic patients reside in the hostels.

It has been traditional in Britain for hospitals to admit all patients referred to them by the general practitioners. The Queen's Park program has established instead a policy of performing pre-admission screening evaluations for all patients referred by the general practitioner. The aim of these evaluations is to identify character disorders, psychopaths, or others considered unsuitable for inpatient treatment. In place of the routine psychiatric admission, an emergency service functions on a 24-hour, seven-day-per-week basis. Patients, usually referred by the general practitioners, are brought into the emergency service by the mental welfare officer. They are seen generally at the rate of two or three per 24-hour period. The availability of this service encourages early referral of psychiatric patients. It is usually possible to treat such patients with drugs, outpatient electro-convulsive therapy, or some other alternative to inpatient hospitalization. Nevertheless, around 700 patients are admitted to the hospital each year, 70% of whom are discharged within a month.

Of course, discharge from the inpatient service is not equivalent to discharge from the psychiatric treatment program. Almost all patients discharged from the inpatient unit continue to be seen on an ambulatory basis as outpatients or in the day hospital where they receive medication, shock therapy, or other treatments.

A number of new patients are seen through domiciliary visits. Such evaluative visits are used especially in the case of geriatric patients. The readiness of the psychiatrist to make diagnostic domiciliary visits has resulted in his being called in much sooner than he had been in former years. The psychiatrist is thus enabled to keep out of the hospital many of the aged who otherwise would "clog up" his beds. Most of the geriatric patients are treated as day patients, residing in the community and brought by local authority ambulances to the hospital's day program as often as seven days per week. Phenothiazines are used liberally with the aged.

Dr. Maurice Silverman, the senior psychiatric consultant in charge of the program, stresses the importance of controlling patients with phenothiazines, which makes it easier for the relatives to manage them at home. The families of the aged therefore demand less frequently that these patients be taken off their hands and hospitalized full-time. In the event of physical illness the aged are quickly given physical examinations, and their somatic needs are looked after. Close attention is given to the maintenance of their nutritional status.

The local authority provides transportation not only for the geriatric patients attending the day care program, but for nearly all day patients as well, regardless of age. This is a highly unusual arrangement, and Dr. Silverman is rather proud of his achievement in bringing this about. He emphasizes the importance of maintaining good community

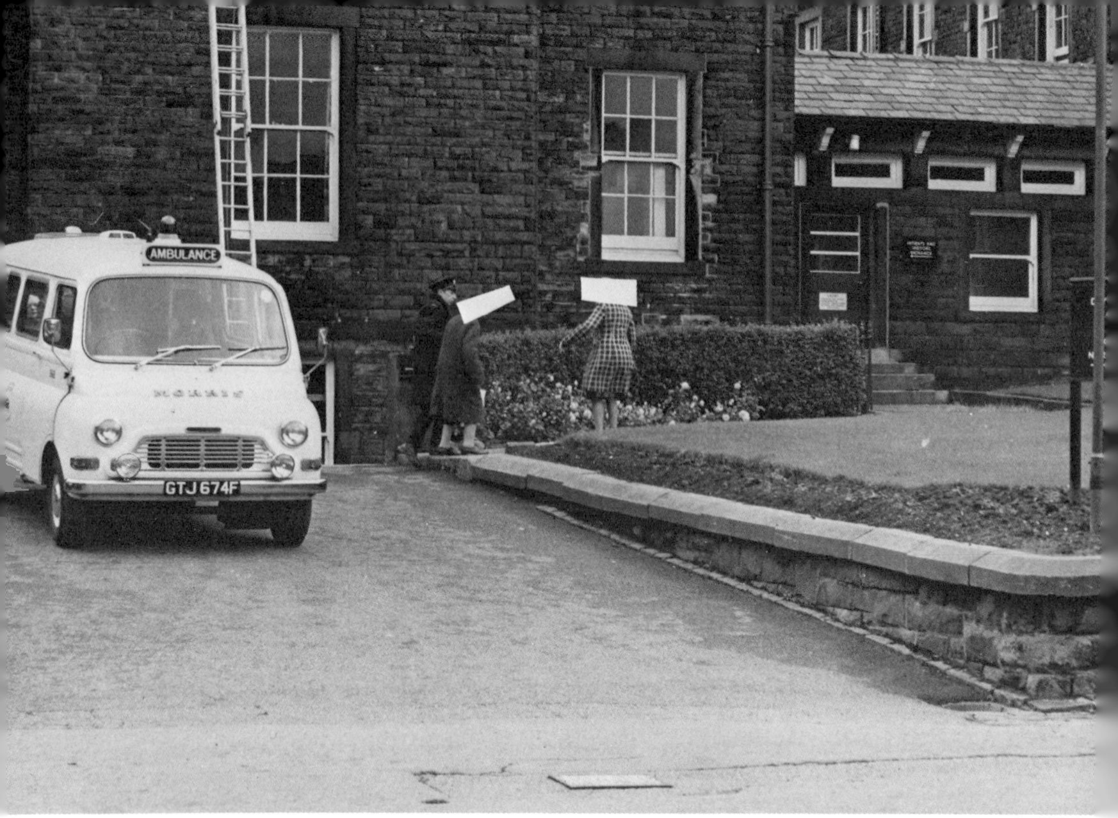

Day patients arriving at the psychiatric unit, Queen's Park Hospital, Blackburn. (*By permission of Mr. H. Harding, Group Secretary, Blackburn and District Hospital Management Committee.*)

relations and demonstrating the significance of his work in order to obtain continued support for his activities.

The Queen's Park Hospital itself consists of a group of old buildings located high atop a hill overlooking the city of Blackburn in the valley below. The psychiatric unit, which is the converted poor-law structure, is a more or less traditionally neat but rather impersonal facility on the hospital grounds. One has the impression of an administrative rather than a clinical interest in patients. The program seems to be considered successful if people are quiet and do not complain. Dealing with aged people has been a continuing problem in Silverman's professional life. He feels that it would be impossible to care for all of the mentally ill of the catchment area without the extensive geriatric service at the hospital, which provides him with relief from the problems of senile and arteriosclerotic patients.

There is no separate day hospital. Ambulant day-patients are managed on the traditional hospital wards; in fact, most of the patients one sees are ambulant and reside in the community. A great deal of electroshock therapy is used on an ambulatory basis. Many patients maintained in the community are followed by their general practitioner with the assistance of periodic checkups made by the mental welfare officer. Silverman maintains a close liaison with the mental welfare officers, the disablement resettlement officer, and the psychologists and social workers of the local authority. He conducts regular conferences with these people to plan the discharge of current inpatients and to discuss problems that have arisen with former inpatients.

Since the implementation of the Seebohm Report, social workers in the Local Authority Health Department, formerly under the jurisdiction of the Medical Officer of Health, are now in a separate department known as the Social Service Department (101). The Director of Social Services, who is a non-medical social worker, is in charge of this new department. The Social Service Department is developing "generic" or non-specialized social workers to take over all social work functions previously assigned to specialized workers of the Welfare Department, Children's Department or Mental Health Department. This of course includes psychiatric social work. In spite of these new developments, however, the psychiatric social workers are still being allowed to maintain joint appointments between the hospital and the new Social Service Department of the local authority.

Silverman works 9/11 time for the Health Service and spends two half-days per week in private practice. There is another psychiatric consultant who comes to Queen's Park two days per week, also two full-time clinical assistants and two registrars, one full-time and one part-time. Silverman's only hospital appointment is at the Queen's Park Hospital; he does not work at any mental hospital.

Queen's Park Hospital is divided into traditional large wards of approximately 14 beds each. There is a good occupational therapy shop with one senior and three basic occupational therapists, and a volunteer worker who teaches pottery. An industrial therapy workshop serves 10-12 male patients, mostly day patients, under the charge of an industrial therapist. This workshop consists chiefly of a machine shop, the emphasis being to move patients into jobs in the community. Some patients, however, remain in the industrial therapy unit for as long as two years. Since the average daily attendance has increased to over 80 patients, the Regional Hospital Board has agreed to substantial extensions for the day-patient occupational therapy and industrial therapy activities.

The dormitory facilities include a male and female admitting ward for the acutely disturbed, suicidal, or other patients requiring close observation; a chronic male and female ward for back-ward patients; and wards for male and female ambulant patients not requiring supervision. All of the wards are unlocked. If it is felt that a patient might run away, he is not given his regular clothes but is dressed in pajamas and dressing gown.

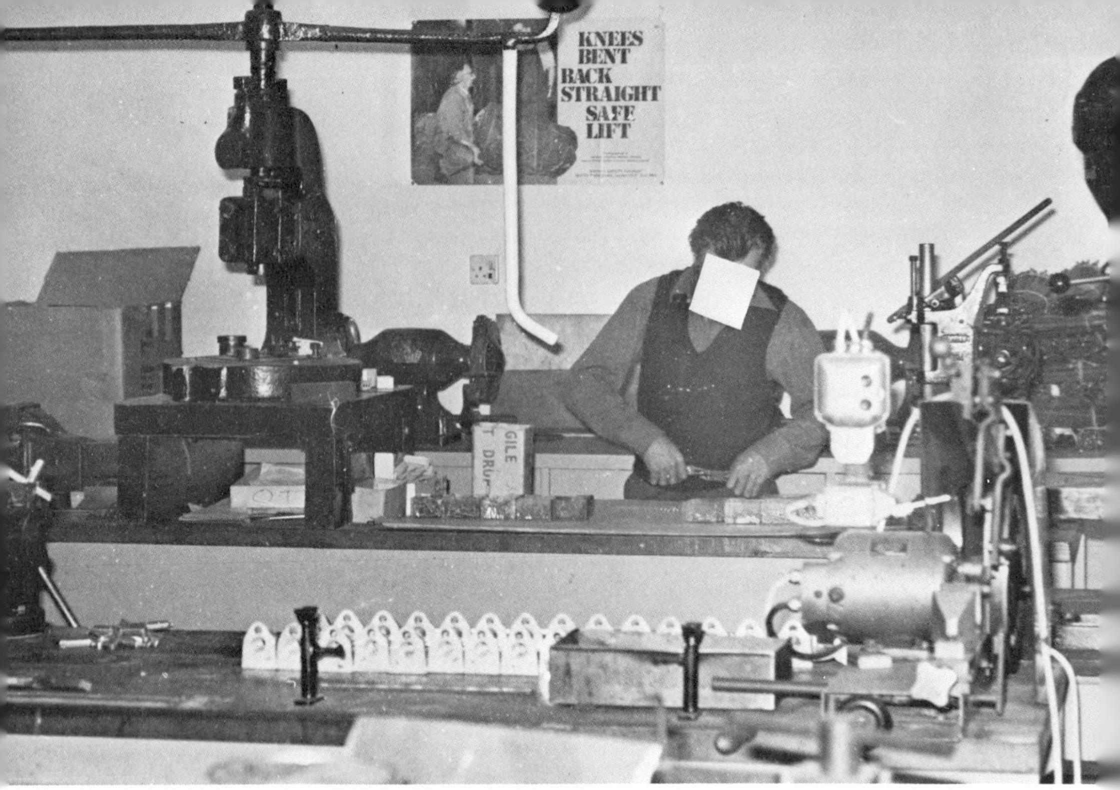

Part of the sheltered industrial workshop, Queen's Park Hospital, Blackburn. (*By permission of Mr. H. Harding, Group Secretary, Blackburn and District Hospital Management Committee.*)

Silverman takes pride in his operation and feels he has made a significant contribution to psychiatric progress. He is pleased that he is frequently visited by outsiders interested in his work and is often asked to speak or write about his service.

SALFORD

Salford, a city of 140,000 in the region of Manchester, is served by two general hospitals, Salford Royal and Hope Hospital, with psychiatric services at the latter, and the Springfield Mental Hospital.

Originally, all general hospital psychiatric services were based at Salford Royal, but all of this activity has now been moved to Hope Hospital, where there is an active outpatient service, a day hospital serving 40-50 patients per day, and an inpatient unit of 30 beds. An additional psychiatric ward is being opened. Hope Hospital is to become an undergraduate teaching hospital, to be renamed the University Hospital of Salford.

At the time of my visit the geriatric service occupied eight beds, and there were 22 psychiatric inpatients. All geriatric patients have since been transferred to a geriatric ward. As I found in many other instances, the geriatric problem is the bane of the psychiatrists, who hope that an active geriatric program will be developed elsewhere to look after the vast majority of aged people. The problem was particularly acute here; before the transfer, the number of geriatric patients on the inpatient unit equalled the number of psychiatric patients.

The situation is now somewhat relieved; however, the dining facilities for the psychiatric patients are adequate only for about 20-25 patients. With the present 30 patients, dining space is crowded. There are plans to convert a storage area into additional dining facilities. The original psychiatric dining facilities were also carved out of an area previously used for storage.

As the limited number of psychiatric beds at Hope Hospital is inadequate for the inpatient needs of the Salford catchment area, the Springfield Mental Hospital continues in use. It regularly cares for approximately 70 or 80 inpatients from the Salford area. The objective of Dr. Hugh Freeman, the senior psychiatric consultant at Salford, is to develop the psychiatric service so that it can care for the entire psychiatric population, and the mental hospital can be dispensed with (29, 30). However, present plans do not include a comprehensive psychiatric unit for patients at Hope Hospital.

In addition to Dr. Freeman, the staff includes another consultant, Dr. Tarsh, and one senior registrar; both Freeman and Tarsh are 9/11 time with the Health Service. There is also a registrar and two part-time assistant psychiatrists, one of whom is trained in psychotherapy. The nursing staff consists of a male nurse in charge (supervisor), plus four sisters (head nurses and assistant head nurses), one staff nurse, four auxiliary nurses (psychiatric aides) and two state enrolled nurses (equivalent of L.P.N.s in the United States who have two years of hospital training and then take a qualifying examination). In the past, the categories of nurses were identified by their respective uniforms, each of which differed significantly from the others, but this is no longer the case. All now wear street clothes on duty.

The facilities at Hope Hospital include a rather large, modern occupational therapy section, which is used as the day hospital unit, and extensive outpatient facilities. The latter encompass the offices of Drs. Freeman and Tarsh, consulting rooms for several social workers, the psychologist's office, the nursing office, and a staff conference room. In addition, in the outpatient section there is an area for administering ambulatory electroshock therapy, plus a recovery room with eight beds.

The outpatient and occupational therapy sections are located on the first floor of the hospital. Upstairs are two conventional hospital wards, one for male and one for female patients. A corridor area has been converted to a day room or television room, utilized by patients of both sexes; in addition there is the previously mentioned dining area, which is very small.

There are four psychiatric social workers who function within the catchment area. Each is appointed half-time by the local authority. Two of the psychiatric social workers also work half-time at Hope Hospital, while the other two are employed at Springfield Hospital. One social worker is assigned to each of the psychiatric consultants at each hospital. In addition, there are some social work students.

According to Freeman, psychiatric emergencies are usually brought to Hope Hospital, although cases of attempted suicide may be taken initially to the Casualty Department at Salford Royal. While there are no psychiatric beds at Salford Royal, psychiatric emergency patients are occasionally kept there overnight and then transferred to Hope Hospital.

The bulk of the clinical work on the psychiatric service is done by the senior registrar, registrar, and assistant psychiatrists. They see the psychiatric emergencies, evaluate all new admissions, and look after the day-to-day management of the patients on the wards. Half of the ward patients are under the supervision of Freeman, the other half under the supervision of Tarsh. Each of them conducts a weekly "ward round" session, at which time the respective patients under the care of each consultant are reviewed with the doctors, social workers, and nurses involved.

At such case conferences or ward rounds, the records of the patients are reviewed briefly, the registrar or nurse comments briefly on the patient's progress or lack of it, or raises questions about particular problems. The social worker adds any comment she may have regarding the family situation. The patient is then usually brought into the conference room for a brief interview with the consultant, who makes a progress note and recommends what the treatment approach should be. The time spent on each case, including patient interview, is between 10 and 15 minutes. Freeman calls this "assembly line psychiatry."

The average length of stay of patients on the inpatient unit is between two and three weeks. Inpatient treatment consists largely of administration of drugs and a great deal of electroshock therapy. Patients are usually continued on a day care or outpatient status following discharge.

An exceptionally close and harmonious relationship is maintained with the local authority services, and the two consultants hold weekly case conferences with the Social Service Department. Before the implementation of the Seebohm Report, 13 social workers of various degrees of qualification were employed by the local authority, of whom six were qualified psychiatric social workers. All of the social workers were appointed mental welfare officers. The senior MWO and his deputy were qualified PSWs. Two of the PSWs maintained joint appointments with the general hospital service, one each assigned respectively to Freeman and Tarsh.

The local authority maintains six day centers, of which four are training centers for the mentally subnormal and two are rehabilitation centers for mental patients. Of the latter, one is for work rehabilitation, and the other is for social rehabilitation of former psychiatric inpatients. Two of the training centers for the mentally subnormal are for children and two for adults. One of the adult subnormal training centers is also used for some chronic schizophrenic patients who require supervision and are not likely to improve.

The Acton Square Industrial Rehabilitation Center is used only for male patients discharged from the mental hospital. The center maintains an industrial therapy unit which performs contract work for local industry, for which patients are paid small amounts of money. The program is geared towards placing patients in jobs in the community.

The other day center, Cleveland House, maintains three programs. One is for aged women who spend their time in occupational therapy activities such as simple handicrafts, which give them a great deal of gratification and sense of accomplishment. Approximately 15 aged women attend each day. They are brought by local authority ambulance, some on a daily basis, others one or more times per week. The second program is also exclusively for women, and was the first day center activity operated by the local authority. Ten to fifteen middle-aged women carry out a variety of occupational therapy activities; they make cushions stuffed with foam rubber, do embroidery, design and carry out cake decoration, or engage in other domestically oriented tasks. The third and most active program is for adolescents of both sexes. Emphasis is placed on social interaction and mutual discussion of problems, although the adolescents do a great deal of acting out. There is a weekly social session and a weekly group therapy session. Each of the three programs meets in a different area of Cleveland House, and each is directed by a different woman leader. None of the leaders has special training for their respective tasks; the woman running the middle-aged group was formerly a physiotherapist for spastic children, and the woman running the group for aged women was formerly a home help. Both seem to possess intuitive resources, are sincerely interested in their charges, and seem to be doing a fine job.

The local authority also operates two hostels, each with 20 beds. Crescent House is chiefly for mentally subnormal adults but also houses a few chronic schizophrenic patients who require maximum assistance and supervision. Kersal House is for former psychiatric inpatients. It is relatively short-stay, with emphasis placed on moving residents into independent living arrangements in the community. A small self-contained flat at Kersal House capable of housing two or three residents is used as a temporary accommodation to establish compatability of residents who might be expected to obtain a flat together in the community. Otherwise, the dormitories consist of bedrooms of three or four beds each, for either males or females. Of the twenty residents, eight are female, twelve male. The warden of the hostel is a young man without special training, very dedicated and bright, who seems to be doing a very good job. He is assisted by his wife, who works in one of the day centers for subnormal children; and by a Ph.D. student, who assists in the supervision of the hostel in return for his room and board. Other student volunteers contribute varying amounts of time to the operation of the hostel. Most of the residents are employed in the community. Each is responsible for his own living area. A cook is employed to provide meals. The social work staff of the local authority provide overall supervision. There are also a number of social clubs for former mental patients, sponsored by the local authority and conducted by the several social workers.

The child guidance clinic is administratively within the Health Department of the local authority, rather than in the Education Department, as is usually the case.

A "general practitioner-social worker team" arrangement involves approximately 12 general practitioners from the community. One, two, or three general practitioners participate in each team, each of which includes a social worker. Some teams include also the midwife, district nurse, health officer, or local authority staff from the Social Service or Education Departments. Each team operates independently, some holding regular meetings, others making different arrangements. These health teams are unique in the area, although analogous programs of somewhat different composition operate rather widely in the vicinity of Coventry.

A psychiatric register of all patients in Salford is funded by the National Department of Health and associated with the Department of Social Medicine and Manchester University. About 1% of the population are in contact with the psychiatric service at all times. Dr. Freeman also conducts studies on "Modecate," a long-acting fluphenazine preparation marketed by Squibb in Britain; he has been collecting data on more than 150 patients who have been on the drug over a three-year period. Freeman also edits the monthly magazine published for the public by the National Association of Mental Health. He has edited several books on community psychiatry and has written extensively on this subject. At the time of my

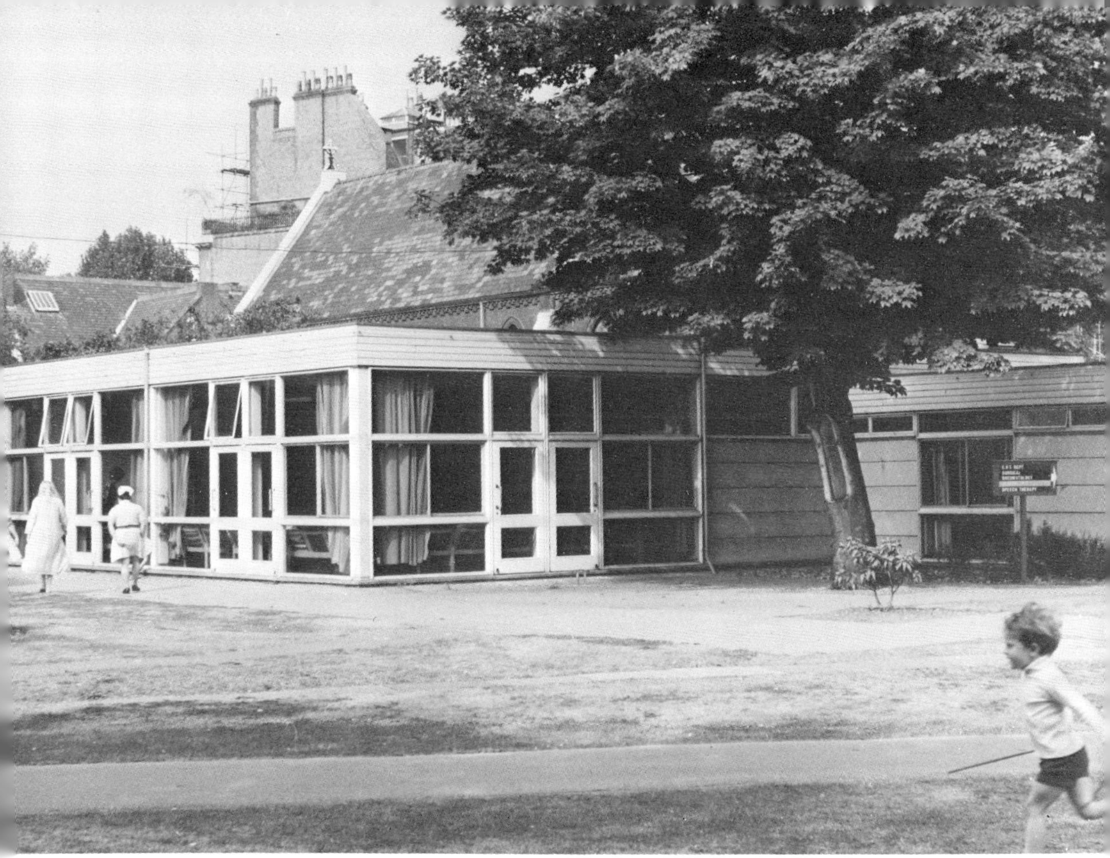

St. Mary Abbots Hospital, London. (*By permission of A.G. King, House Governor, St. Mary Abbots Hospital.*)

visit he was about to make a lecture trip to the United States, sponsored partially by Squibb.

ST. MARY ABBOTS HOSPITAL

St. Mary Abbots Hospital is a Victorian general hospital serving the Borough of Kensington and Chelsea in London. As a result of the bombing during World War II, some of the hospital buildings were leveled, and for a time, the grounds surrounding the remaining buildings were covered with lawn and flowers. Several years ago Dr. A. A. Baker, then psychiatric consultant to St. Mary Abbots but subsequently promoted to the Health Ministry, prevailed upon the administration to utilize some of this space for the construction of a psychiatric inpatient unit. Prior to that time a psychiatric outpatient clinic had been functioning at St. Mary Abbots, operated by consultants from the Banstead Mental Hospital.

A group consisting of Dr. Baker, Mr. King, the hospital administrator, an architect, the chief surgeon, and some other consultants formed a committee to plan the psychiatric unit. The unit is built of prefabricated materials customarily used for the construction of schools, and is rather flimsy. Its shape was somewhat determined by the presence on the hospital grounds of a good-sized church, so that the psychiatric unit sort of surrounds the church on three sides. The one-story unit has six 6-bedded wards and 4 single rooms, a large dining area, and an adjacent sizeable day room. Baker included a room for the care of infants whose mothers might need psychiatric hospitalization (4). There is a utility room which is actually used by the nursing staff to store medications, particularly Modecate, which is widely used. There is a room for administration of electroshock therapy, four or five consulting rooms, a small nursing office, a patients' kitchen area, and several alcoves which can be used for waiting rooms or visiting areas. The ward population is comprised of 26 women and 14 men.

The medical staff consists of two consultants (Dr. M. S. DeMowbray and Dr. Rohde), two medical assistants (one assigned to each consultant), and three registrars (one and a half assigned to each consultant). The consultants and medical assistants spend three days per week at the St. Mary Abbots Psychiatric Unit and two and one-half days weekly at the Banstead Hospital. The registrars are full time at St. Mary Abbots. There is one psychologist and one social worker, a nursing staff of 30, almost all of whom are senior nurses, and three occupational therapists. At present there is one part-time senior social worker and one full-time social work assistant, but Dr. DeMowbray, the senior consultant, regards this number as inadequate.

A busy psychiatric outpatient clinic is operated in the psychiatric unit, the consultants taking turns in conducting the clinic. Each may see as many as five new patients per day. Some may have been referred by their general practitioner for evaluation of a psychiatric complaint, for determination of the ultimate disposition, or for treatment; or others may have been referred from another service of the hospital for an evaluation and report. An average of 5-10 patients per week are referred by the Department of Gynecology for a psychiatric opinion regarding indications for abortions, but this number has been decreasing. The other outpatients seen are post-discharge follow-up cases, and several psychotherapy cases are seen by the consultant each day he is on duty. In addition, a large number of patients return for their regular Modecate injection, administered by the nurses. There is a record room and secretarial office, where the two secretaries keep track of the patients and perform secretarial duties for the medical staff. A full-time receptionist handles clerical work, telephone calls, and appointments.

In addition to the inpatient service, there is a day hospital in another part of the hospital grounds. This was originally an unused facility resembling a storage area. The roof was in bad shape and the walls in need of repair. The psychiatric department renovated the structure and established a good-sized occupational therapy area, an office for the occupational therapists, and a small reading or music room. There is also a beauty room and space for storage of supplies. This area accommodates as many as 50 day patients, although it is fairly crowded with this number. The average daily number of patients in attendance is 40. Only two nurses are assigned to the day hospital, in addition to the three occupational therapists. There were 5,748 attendances during 1968-69, of which 1,452 were by male patients and 4,296 by female patients. During 1968, 41 patients attending the day hospital had to be readmitted as inpatients.

The ages of the patients range from 18 to over 80. A number of day hospital patients are rather chronic and continue their attendance indefinitely. Other patients stay an average of 8-12 weeks in the day hospital. Patients may be admitted to the day hospital following discharge from the inpatient unit or directly from the outpatient clinic.

The only types of patients not accepted for day hospital treatment are drug addicts and aggressive psychopaths. The London ambulance service provides transportation for the patients if required. Failure of a patient to turn up for a scheduled day hospital session is investigated by a member of the nursing staff, who makes a domiciliary visit.

The activities of the day hospital include light industrial work, clerical work, printing, cookery, domestic activities, carpentry, dressmaking and other activities. There are also recreational and social events, which include outings to local places of interest, play-reading, music, group games, etc. Most patients are on chemotherapy of some sort. Patients in the day hospital who require electroconvulsive therapy (ECT) receive this in the ECT area of the inpatient unit. ECT is also given to outpatients. The day hospital patients take their meals in the dining room of the inpatient unit at a second sitting for lunch. The day hospital is also used by inpatients for occupational therapy activities.

Regular group psychotherapy sessions are held. In recent years, there has been a great expansion in the use of group meetings, both in the inpatient unit and at the day hospital. Staff, as well as patients, participate. This development has been stimulated by Rohde and DeMowbray, both of whom are interested in psychotherapy. The aim has been to form a therapeutic community, seeking improved communication and mutual understanding between staff and patients.

In the inpatient unit each consultant now holds two weekly meetings for the patients under his care. These meetings are attended by junior medical staff and some of the nurses and are followed by short discussion groups for staff alone. A patient's suggestion box has been instituted. These suggestions are discussed in the whole-unit meetings conducted by the nursing staff.

The psychiatric unit serves a catchment area population of approximately 130,000 from four postal districts of the borough (S.W. 5, S.W. 7, W. 8, and W. 14). Some patients from S.W. 3, S.W. 6, and S.W. 10 also attend the day hospital, but admission to the inpatient service is fairly well confined to patients residing in the first four postal districts. The clinical firms are organized along catchment area lines. Rohde assumes responsibility for patients from S.W. 5 and S.W. 7, while DeMowbray supervises the treatment of patients from W. 8 and W. 14. If a general practitioner from these areas requires the assistance of a psychiatrist, he has no choice of consultant. If the case is from DeMowbray's area, he is the one who is called, while Rohde is called if the patient resides in his area. Patients may be admitted by other members of the staff on an emergency basis, depending upon who is on duty, but responsibility for the supervision of treatment in the hospital belongs to the consultant in charge of the area whence the patient comes. Patients from outside the catchment area are referred elsewhere.

St. Mary Abbots has referred very few patients to Banstead Mental Hospital. Through its inpatient, outpatient, and day hospital activities, it has been able to treat all comers without regard to the nature of the behavior disorder or diagnosis. The patients are frequently brought in by the police and merely dumped on the doorstep, and include addicts, drunks, and other problem patients. The majority of patients, however, are referred by the general practitioner. A significant percentage of the patients admitted to the psychiatric unit of St. Mary Abbots are transients, largely foreign nationals from every European country, the United States, and several Asian countries. These patients are mostly young people who arrive at the West London Air Terminal, which is in the catchment area, and find lodgings at one of the many small hostels in the area. Some of them are already psychotic when they get off the plane. Such patients are brought to the hospital by the police; emergency treatment is provided free to foreign nationals by the Health Service. One patient has returned to London five times with a psychotic break each time and has been hospitalized in each instance at St. Mary Abbots.

Most of the day-to-day care is of course handled by the registrar. Since the registrars are full-time at St. Mary Abbots, there are no registrars of these firms at Banstead Hospital. As a consequence, the consultants must do more of the detail work with their patients at the mental hospital than their counterparts. Rohde and DeMowbray together make up one of the consultant firms at Banstead. There are a number of other consultant firms as well, not connected with any general hospital. They are nevertheless responsible for particular catchment areas around London, and if their patients require admission they must be sent to Banstead. For a long time there was no need to admit patients to Banstead from the catchment area covered by the St. Mary Abbots. Consequently, the population of the DeMowbray-Rohde firm at Banstead decreased at a rate of 100 per year. Recently, the number of beds at St. Mary Abbots became inadequate, so that there is now some spill-over of admissions into Banstead, and their population is no longer declining.

Rohde and DeMowbray feel they have by this time discharged from Banstead just about every patient who has any potential for success in the community and that the remainder of their patients at Banstead represent the rock-bottom who will have to remain in the hospital probably until they die. For the most part they are chronic schizophrenic patients who have become senile. These psychiatrists feel that the accumulation of long-stay chronic hospital patients can be fully avoided through the method of rapid, early, vigorous treatment in the general hospital psychiatric unit. They consider that Modecate has contributed greatly to the success of this treatment approach.

In 1967, there were 435 admissions to and 429 discharges from St. Mary Abbots' Psychiatric Unit, and in 1968, 520 admissions and 520 discharges; 1,605 outpatients were seen in 1967 and 1,720 in 1968. The average length of stay in 1967 was 19.6 days; this was reduced to 15.5 days in 1968. Around 30% of admissions are on legal orders of some kind. In 1967, 29% of the patients admitted were readmissions; in 1968 this figure was 32%.

The psychiatrists regard readmission of patients as part of the natural course of events when dealing with chronic psychiatric illness. They are not concerned about a "revolving door" problem. Rather they believe that several brief admissions to the general hospital unit obviate the need for longer periods as an inpatient in the mental hospital. The patient therefore spends more of his lifetime as a functioning member of the community and avoids the debilitating consequences of institutionalization.

The relationship with the other specialties of the general hospital is fairly good, chiefly as a result of a vigorous public relations effort made by Dr. Baker when the unit first opened. Nevertheless, there is still a considerable residual attitude of suspicion on the part of the other physicians towards psychiatry. There is a fairly close working relationship in cases calling for joint responsibility, such as overdoses or post-partum psychosis. Medical care is readily available for patients in the psychiatric unit, and the psychiatric unit gives prompt service to patients elsewhere in the hospital requiring psychiatric attention.

St. Stephens, another large general hospital in the Chelsea/Kensington group, is planning a significant new addition. The psychiatrists are fearful that on its completion a percentage of the medical and surgical activity of St. Mary Abbots will be moved to St. Stephens, the psychiatric service at St. Mary Abbots will be significantly expanded, and a geriatric program will likewise be introduced. This prospect could change St. Mary Abbots from an acute general hospital to a chronic geriatric and psychiatric hospital and is something the psychiatrists would like very much to avoid. They see it as a reflection of the still rather primitive attitude of the non-psychiatric physicians towards psychiatry and mental illness.

At Fulham there is another general hospital psychiatric unit quite similar to the one at St. Mary Abbots, staffed by consultants from the Longrove Mental Hospital. These psychiatrists, in contrast to those at St. Mary Abbots, use the general hospital unit only for the short-term intensive treatment of acute psychiatric cases, neurotics, or acute psychotic episodes and continue to send the chronic or long-stay patients to the mental hospital. Their philosophy is at the other extreme from that characterizing the St. Mary Abbots Hospital, which reflects the attitude of Baker. The St. Mary Abbots psychiatrists are skeptical of the Fulham approach but have adopted a wait-and-see attitude.

The program of admitting infants with their psychiatrically ill mothers was a pet approach of Dr. Baker's (4). However, the facility at the psychiatric unit of St. Mary Abbots is really not adequate to care for these infants. Consequently mothers with post-partum psychosis are customarily addmitted to Banstead Hospital, together with their infants, where a more suitable unit has been established by the medical assistant, Dr. Morrison, who has worked with Baker for a number of years.

During my visit I met an architect who was drawing plans for a standard design for psychiatric units to be developed at general hospitals throughout Britain. This approach has been given support by the Ministry of Health at Baker's urging. The basic unit has two stories. On one side is a 30-bed ward and above that another 30-bed ward. On the other side of the first floor is a day hospital, and the second floor consists of consulting rooms, record rooms, electroshock therapy area, etc., to provide facilities for outpatients, inpatients, and day patients seen by the medical staff. The architect was visiting various hospitals to get ideas before finalizing the plans. This program seems to represent the current direction of the Ministry of Health in developing community psychiatry programs. The main effect of the emphasis upon general hospitals is to shift the therapeutic effort from the tail end (i.e., rehabilitation of the chronic hospitalized patient) to the input end, hopefully preventing the accumulation of chronic long-stay patients in mental institutions. A recent directive from the Health Ministry looks towards a more or less complete transfer of responsibility for providing psychiatric inpatient treatment from the mental institutions to general hospital psychiatric units (42).

11

Specialized voluntary programs

Voluntary organizations are a traditional feature of British life. Most social reforms over the past several centuries were originated by groups of interested citizens who banded together and pooled their resources in support of the particular causes in which they believed. The flourishing of voluntary organizations during the last half of the 19th century and the first half of the 20th century helped to stimulate the participation of the government in health and social welfare.

Now that the state has assumed wide responsibility for meeting social and health needs, one might have expected a decline in the activities of the voluntary organizations. On the contrary, the number of organizations and the scope of their activities have continued to increase since World War II. The major change is that now the voluntary organizations work in close cooperation with national and local governmental agencies, and the state services often work through the voluntary societies. While the voluntary groups continue to receive substantial support from voluntary sources, grants from local and central government support increasing portions of the budgets. Voluntary financial contributions come from organizations as well as individuals. These organizations include industrial and commercial firms and large charitable trusts. Among the more important in the latter group are: the Calouste Gulbenkian Foundation, the Nuffield Foundation, and the Wolfson Foundation, as well as the Carnegie United Kingdom Trust and King George's Jubilee Trust.

The number of voluntary organizations now runs into the thousands, ranging from large national organizations to small local groups. Their functions vary widely, ranging from religious, humanitarian, and political objectives, to various aspects of health, education, and welfare. Among the national organizations relevant to mental health are: the Mental After-Care Association; the National Association for Mental Health; the National Association of Leagues of Hospital Friends; the National Society for Mentally Handicapped Children; the National Marriage Guidance Council; and the National Council of Social Service. These and related organizations function in ways similar to their American counterparts.

Another type of voluntary organization is the self-help or membership group. In such organizations people sharing a common problem or affliction band together to take action for their mutual benefit. Thus there are, for example, the British Limbless ex-Servicemen's Association, the British Polio Fellowship, the Consumers' Council, the Haemophilia Society, etc. Among those of interest to psychiatrists are the Therapeutic Social Clubs. These groups, made up of former mental patients, usually with some professional leadership, are autonomous local chapters, often related to a particular hospital. The members are "graduates," and the group is usually named for the day of the week on which they meet.

In this section will be described a voluntary assistance service (the Citizens' Advice Bureau); a half-way house program (Richmond Fellowship); and a therapeutic social club (the Friday Evening Club).

CITIZENS' ADVICE BUREAUX

Citizens' Advice Bureaux (CABs) had their start in 1939 as a wartime advice and information service. The movement has developed into one of Britain's largest voluntary undertakings. There are now approximately 500 bureaux in operation, helping individuals to benefit from the various services available to them and interpreting the law to citizens who have difficulty in understanding it. The CABs have remained an independent source of advice and assistance while the government has been increasing its health and welfare responsibility.

The independence of the CAB from government is particularly important, as the CABs are often involved with citizens' complaints about local authorities. The CAB tries to maintain objectivity rather than identify with the complainant, and sometimes its role is to help the individual accept an adverse government decision. But its readiness to promote the cause of the individual, if the government is in error or is unfair, enables the citizen to trust the CAB even when it sides with the government. Thus it is in a position to clarify misunderstandings and ease tensions, by relieving the person's feelings that he has been treated unjustly.

The coordinating body of the bureaux is the National Citizens' Advice Bureau Council, supported in part by a grant from the central government. In London the bureaux are affiliated with the various Borough Councils of Social Service, which take responsibility for their support, staffing, and operation. Most bureaux receive some financial subsidy from the local authorities. Staffing varies widely; leadership staff are usually paid social workers while the majority of other staff are specially selected, trained volunteers.

The Camden Council of Social Service operates five Citizens' Advice Bureaux located in various parts of the borough (West Hampton, East Hampton, Kings Cross, Kentish Town, and Swiss Cottage) (92). Each is staffed by part-time, trained social workers and volunteers. In each office the time put in by the part-time social workers adds up to something over one full-time worker, although the precise amount of professional times varies between the offices, depending on the volume of activity.

The volunteers are carefully selected from among the many applicants to the Camden Council of Social Service for volunteer assignments. Two major criteria are used in the selection process: intelligence and scholastic ability, including the capacity for independent reading and handling of sometimes complex paper work; and the personality characteristics that would enable them to work with people with problems, without themselves becoming depressed or otherwise emotionally disturbed. Thus, the CAB volunteers tend to be better educated and more stable emotionally than the usual volunteer worker. Nevertheless, occasional errors in selection have been made.

A candidate for a volunteer position is generally assigned to observe the activities of the CAB for a period of about one month. During that time the candidate is likewise under observation and continues to be evaluated for suitability. Candidates found unsuitable to serve as CAB volunteers are generally assigned to some other activity operated by the Camden Council of Social Service. Once selected, Citizens' Advice Bureau workers are carefully trained.

The activities of the Camden CABs are funded entirely by the local authority. Although it pays the rent and salaries and provides the supplies, the local authority refrains from trying to influence the policies of the CAB. However, there are representatives from the local authority on the governing board of the Council of Social Services.

The Citizens' Advice Bureaux are well-established units known throughout the community and used by all classes of citizens. Some people come just to have someone they can gripe to about their problems, not really expecting nor even necessarily wanting anything in particular to be done about them. Nevertheless, the worker may find some area where she can be helpful, even regarding such "gripes."

Sometimes the citizen is concerned about a trivial matter, but the worker finds a more complex and serious problem when hearing the person out. Thus, many otherwise unrecognized needs are discovered. While this function of the CAB is not regarded by them as a mental health one, it is clear that both the ventilation aspect and the help given to cope with crisis situations fit into the "primary prevention" model.

Additionally, the contribution which the CABs make to strengthening family life, as well as steering people to supportive social services in the community, helps to relieve some of the community pressures generated by the increasing emphasis on community care for psychiatric patients.

Beyond this, they give direct aid to citizens with legitimate complaints. This may be administrative help in getting claims adjusted or processed, à la "Action Line," or direct intervention on the citizen's behalf before the local "administrative tribunal," an agency of the national "Council of Tribunals," which attempts to standardize administrative practice and is not a legal body like a court.

Conversely, CABs also serve to interpret government jargon to the citizen. They thus serve an interpretive role in both directions and also serve as feedback to the government agencies regarding the reaction of the public to government policies.

Another function of the CAB is public education. For example, they have put out a booklet on buying and renting a house to help people learn how to go about this activity, so very important in British life. Housing is a major problem, and this booklet helps people avoid pitfalls involved in trying to cope with it. Also, while the CABs do not regard themselves as mental health agencies, they nevertheless found themselves consulted with increasing frequency on mental health problems as the emphasis on community mental health increased. So they put out a booklet "The Citizen and Mental Care," a summary of the Mental Health Act of 1959, its mode of operation, and a delineation of the rights of mental patients (31).

The CAB is also active in consumer protection. For example, in the government's effort to combat air pollution, some pollution-producing fuels were outlawed in many areas. The need to change to new fuels usually required mandatory conversion of heating equipment, for which the government reimburses the citizen, provided prior permission is obtained. A number of unscrupulous salesmen of inferior equipment, for which reimbursement was not awarded, tried to high-pressure people into contracting for such equipment without going to the local authority first. The CABs disseminated warnings about this practice, telling people of their rights and advising the proper procedures to follow in order to obtain compensation. They also give advice on "hire-purchase" schemes (installment buying).

In the Camden CABs, the most frequent inquiries relate to property and land, followed by requests for information on civic, local, and national services, and for assistance with family and personal problems. Then come questions relating to employment, consumer matters, social security, health and medical questions, education and training, communication and travel, taxes, and insurance.

In Camden many CAB clients, by virtue of limited intelligence, education, or cultural background, are ill equipped to solve the problems arising from the complexities of modern living, especially those relating to coping with the programs of the welfare state. The aid offered by the Citizens' Advice Bureau is limited to those areas specifically requested by the client, even though the worker may discover other areas of difficulty of which the client himself is not yet aware. In the course of work with clients, however, opportunities often present themselves for the worker to bring such additional problems to the attention of the client so that he may be helped with these as well. Such initially unrecognized problems often include mental or emotional difficulties. When overt psychiatric problems are discovered, the CAB worker will attempt to refer the client to an appropriate mental health agency.

In addition to their more routine activities, the Camden Citizens' Advice Bureaux continually explore new ways in which their agency can become more effective. As a consequence, they have embarked on a number of experimental ventures. For example, in 1968-69 the CAB experimented in the use of workers in a Magistrate's court. In addition, the CAB set up a "Neighborhood Center" as a focus for community organization and action in a "tower block" of new residents made up of diverse groups of people displaced from their former decrepit abodes, which had been torn down.

Other experiments conducted by the Camden CAB have related to statutory legal aid and advice services (they set up a program for clients to talk to volunteer lawyers about their problems), an attempt to place a Greek-speaking worker in the Kentish town office to deal with numerous Cypriot immigrants who did not speak English, and setting up at the Swiss Cottage office a service to help the bereaved, operated under the guidance of Dr. C. Murray Parkes of the Tavistock Centre.

The Camden Bureaux believe that their experiments have demonstrated how each bureau can offer a very personal service, most meaningful for its particular clientele.

RICHMOND FELLOWSHIP HOUSE, KENSINGTON

The Richmond Fellowship began as an experiment in 1959, when Miss Elly Jansen attempted to develop a half-way house with a psychiatric orientation. She did not have definite guidelines at the outset, but sought to avoid both the authoritarian model and the self-government model. She believed that the authoritarian approach was impersonal and repressive, did not permit emotional expression and conflict, and tended to regiment and institutionalize patients; on the other hand she felt that the over-permissive, self-government model considered everything therapeutic, placed patients at the mercy of the most disturbed members of the group, often demonstrated an antiprofessional bias, and emphasized a "moral therapy" or even religious orientation.

Miss Jansen learned as she worked, but her efforts were so successful that within a few months the applications outnumbered the places available. Rather than attempt to expand the program piecemeal, Miss Jansen decided to set up an organization which could raise the necessary funds to purchase properties, negotiate with the authorities, recruit a trained staff, and conduct research. There are 18 Richmond Fellowship Houses throughout England (61). Although all of the houses have the same basic structure and orientation, and the staff encounter the same problems, each house has its own individual character.

Other developments soon followed. The requirements for staff training resulted in the development of a full-scale college. The success of the program in England led to the export of the idea to the United States. The Richmond Fellowship of America was incorporated in 1968, and several half-way houses have been developed under its auspices. In 1970, this program was also introduced in Australia, and there are plans to establish additional experimental units in Italy and Israel.

Applications for admission to fellowship houses are submitted by psychiatrists, psychoanalysts, general practitioners, clergy, mental health departments, relatives, and friends in behalf of the mentally ill patients. Whatever the referral source, the patient must be recommended by a psychiatrist and remain under his direct supervision while staying in the Fellowship House. Men and women between 16 and 65 years of age are eligible, but most residents fall between the ages of 20 and 40. Most of the residents have high intelligence and good educational background.

The Richmond Fellowship Houses are supported by fees paid by the residents, either from private funds or by means of a subsidy from the local authority responsible for their care. During 1966-67, patients from 65 hospitals were accepted as residents of the various houses, and their fees were paid by 45 different local authorities. (This does not include those paying privately.) In addition to income from residents' fees, the fellowship receives grants from various sources, including private foundations, local governments, and industry, in support of a number of specific projects.

The houses provide places for approximately 280 patients (61). Various houses have specialized clienteles. Thus, the Southhampton House provides lodging for adolescent girls; ex-alcoholics reside at the Purley House; the Havering House accommodates mothers with young children; and a new house at Oxford serves the undergraduate students. The original Richmond Fellowship House is used for long-term schizophrenics, as is the house at Swiss Cottage; the one at St. John's Wood provides for a mixed group of younger patients. Denbridge is the training house, where there are 20 residents and a warden who is also a tutor. People who are preparing to become wardens spend two months at the Denbridge House in training.

A number of the houses have a mixed group of patients, and this is the case with the Richmond Fellowship House at Kensington, which I visited.

The house is located in a middle-class residential area, a short distance from Kensington High Street, one of London's major shopping centers. Not identifably different from its neighbors on either side, it looks old but not particularly run-down.

The building has four stories, the top floor serving as living quarters for the warden and his wife. Living quarters for the residents are on the second and third floors, with a toilet and bath on the landing between each floor. On the first floor is a lounge for the residents and additional living quarters; on the ground floor or basement level there is an all-purpose recreation room, a dining room, the kitchen used for preparing the residents' meals, and another office for the warden. Most of the rooms are either two- or three-bed rooms. A few are single rooms, one of which is occupied by the bursar and another by one of the female residents. The rooms are nicely but not elaborately furnished, and many of the items in them are the personal possessions of the residents. At the time of my visit, remodeling was in progress on the basement level, where a new laundry facility was being built and some plumbing repairs were being made.

The Kensington House is approved for 11 residents, although there are potential beds for 14. At the time of my visit only 6 residents occupied the building: 4 women and 2 men. Ultimately, it was expected that Kensington House would house 8 women and 6 men, but it had not yet had more than 10 residents living at the hostel at a given time.

The age of the residents at the time of my visit ranged from 23 to 40 years. The Kensington House tends to attract young, intelligent patients who have a need to be close to central London. The makeup of the population is maintained by a selection procedure, whereby following familiarization with the background of the applicant and a meeting with him, the current residents vote whether or not to accept him. In addition, the warden may refuse to accept any potential resident who he feels will not benefit from the setting or not fit in with the other residents.

Most of the houses are bigger than the one in Kensington; the usual number of residents is 20 to 30 per house. Although the Kensington House is only partly occupied, the fellowship is building another training house nearby at Nottinghill Gate, where they already maintain a "three-fourth house" (in contrast to a "half-way house"), consisting of two flats, one for men, the other for women, with no supervision of any kind.

Supervision at the Kensington House is provided by the warden and his wife (Mr. and Mrs. Ford), and a bursar. The warden is a gray-haired man in his fifties, formerly a priest. His wife, in her forties, was formerly a speech therapist. They seemed an ideal pair for the kind of work they do. The previous warden at Kensington House had been a young, unmarried girl, younger than many of the residents, and when the present warden and his wife came to the house some residents resented trading a peer figure for a parental figure. After several months, however, the Fords made a satisfactory adjustment to the residents, and the residents accepted the Fords. The bursar also seems to get along and fit in well with the resident group. He had only been there for three months at the time of my visit and was himself in training as a bursar. The man he had replaced was completely untrained and left to acquire the proper training.

Most residents are occupied during the day. Two were in psychoanalysis, and the others were working or attending school. Most residents who leave the house go on to better things, but a few return to the house. The average length of stay at Kensington House is about 18 months.

Mr. Ford told me that the six current residents had paired off into two sets of triangles which were in some conflict with each other, although the Fords seemed to feel that this friction was becoming less intense. There did not seem to be any particular specific program or overall approach, other than the general principles laid down by Elly Jansen; nevertheless, the place seemed to be fairly well run and smoothly operating.

The residents seemed fairly congenial. There are regular weekly group meetings to discuss their relationships, and additional ones are called as needed. The residents talk out their interpersonal problems at length. They also use the meetings to discuss the operational problems of the house. In addition, the residents often consult individually with the warden or his wife regarding personal problems that they may have.

Housekeeping is shared among the residents, and the warden, his wife, and the bursar help out. One of the women residents, in analysis but not working, was currently doing the cooking, with the assistance of the warden and his wife. The residents contribute to the cost of food, decisions are made collectively as to what will be purchased, and one or another resident is assigned to do the weekly marketing. The house operates on a strict budget.

THE FRIDAY EVENING CLUB

Although retired from his responsibilities at the Marlborough Day Hospital, Dr. Joshua Bierer has remained actively involved with another of his creations, the therapeutic social club. He continues to attend and work with a group of independent clubs for former psychiatric patients. These clubs meet in the evenings one each weekday at various locations around London.

Dr. Bierer first became interested in the community approach to psychiatric treatment in 1938, and over the years he has been responsible for a number of therapeutic innovations. Although his novel ideas were not immediately appreciated by his institutionally oriented colleagues, many of his pioneer contributions have been widely emulated since interest in the community approach has become more general. One of his earliest emphases was on increased patient participation in the treatment process. This idea led logically to the notions of the therapeutic community and patient self-government. Thus, when Bierer developed the first social clubs to meet the re-socialization needs of socially isolated former mental patients, it was natural that he organized the clubs along the lines of self-government.

Several therapeutic social clubs were established by Bierer specifically for former patients of the Marlborough Day Hospital. However, he recognized the need quite early for such programs for patients from other hospitals and therefore, also established a number of independent clubs. He continues to attend almost every meeting of these clubs, although there is also a staff of several social workers who are present.

The membership is made up of former mental hospital patients from a number of institutions. Some individuals have been members for as long as 20 years, during which time Bierer has had an excellent opportunity for longitudinal follow-up studies of the effectiveness of this approach.

I attended with Bierer a meeting of the Friday Night Club. It was held in an old but richly furnished house, the home of a former mental patient who had been leucotomized. The patient hostess is quite wealthy by inheritance, and several years ago offered her house as a meeting place when the usual meeting place of the Friday Night Club was no longer available. Since there are many disturbed and antisocial patients in the club, Bierer at first hesitated, fearing that some of the furnishings of the house might become damaged or that some of the valuable pieces might be stolen. Finally, however, he decided to risk it. It proved to be a wise decision. The club has been meeting regularly at this house every Friday night ever since, with no untoward consequences.

While driving to the meeting in Bierer's car, we encountered two patients walking along the street who were also going to the meeting, and Bierer offered them a lift. One of them first had to take supper to her husband, who works as a ticket agent in the underground. Bierer therefore drove her to the underground station first, and then we all proceeded to the club meeting. Along the way both members extolled the values of the club to their own mental well-being.

When we arrived at the house, the meeting was already in progress. A patient was complaining that he had attended a dance and someone had refused to dance with him. His reactions to the situation were quite paranoid, and other patients were trying to help him adjust to his feelings of rejection by recounting their own experiences. Generally, they were quite supportive and understanding.

Because of this tendency of the patients to be actively "therapeutic" with one another, Bierer had told me that it would be difficult to distinguish which were the social workers and which were the patients in the group. I did not find this difficult. Not only were the social workers obviously "professional" in their approach to the patients, but the patients tended to give the workers' comments a deference which was not given to remarks made by other patients. Furthermore, many of the patients were obviously *patients*; that is, they appeared unkempt or disheveled, stared vacantly, or exhibited evidence of mental deterioration. Many appeared quite withdrawn, and a few were definitely bizarre.

Shortly after we arrived, Bierer interrupted the discussion centering around the young man and turned his attention to another member of the club who was the only American in the group. Apparently, there had been some problems brought to Bierer's attention with which he now meant to confront this man. He first asked the patient's permission to discuss the matter before the group, and the patient agreed.

The confrontation related to an outing the American had made with another group member to spend a weekend with the brother and sister-in-law of the latter, who lived in the country. Apparently, this patient's brother had called Bierer to complain about the young American's behavior on that occasion. The other patient had evidently become acutely disturbed over the weekend and had to be rehospitalized, much to the concern of his brother.

Bierer began to interrogate the American in a challenging tone, inquiring whether he was aware of any misbehavior on his part during the weekend. At this the group as a whole, including the social workers, took exception. They felt that Bierer was attacking the patient before the group, and several expressed the idea that such matters might best be discussed privately. It was clear that many in the group were made uncomfortable by the encounter, and because Bierer was the "attacker," they tended to side at this point with the patient.

Bierer pointed out that he had asked the patient's permission before raising the issue in the group, and that the patient had consented. Nevertheless, he subsequently softened his tone of voice and spoke less sharply to the American. As the meeting continued and more details of the events of the weekend became known to the members of the group, they later seemed less sympathetic towards the American, although they continued to remain friendly and supportive and tried to be helpful.

The patient had acknowledged that he made a number of telephone calls to the United States, using the telephone of the other patient's brother. As the American responded to Bierer's questions, it became apparent that the telephone calls had been made in the middle of the night; that they required the operator to call back after the calls had been placed, resulting in the telephone ringing and waking the household; and that while the American had asked and received permission to use the telephone, he had not made it clear what the destination of the calls was to be. While the American readily acknowledged telephoning, he did not indicate at the beginning how many calls he had placed. He insisted, however, that he had asked to be given a tabulation of the charges by the operator, and before leaving repaid his friend's brother for the full amount of the calls. The brother had told Bierer, however, that he had not been adequately compensated.

The brother had also complained that the American had been under the influence of alcohol and that he had pressured the other patient into drinking to excess. The brother believed that it was this fact that had precipitated the breakdown which had necessitated rehospitalization. The American claimed that he had, indeed, had some "apple wine," which he had brought into the house only with the permission of the brother and that he had been careful not to drink too much. He insisted that he had not been inebriated and said that the brother already had a larger bottle of the same wine in the house.

As the discussion developed it became clear that the American could not be completely forthright in his description of his own behavior, even though he gave a great show of doing so. It also seemed likely that part of the difficulty lay with the brother, who had been disturbed by the patient's decompensation, as well as by the American's insensitive and un-English behavior.

The various members tried to point out to the American that he had exercised extremely poor judgment from the beginning. They attempted to explain what the expectations of proper English families would be under the circumstances and how this would differ from what the American might have anticipated. Despite his apparent acceptance of the comments of his fellow group members, this part of the meeting concluded without any definite decisions being made. The American expressed his willingness to continue to explore the matter with Bierer.

Bierer later explained that his confrontation of the patient was not typical of his usual participation in the group. He confided that he had felt it necessary to intervene in this manner on this occasion because he was concerned about the American's behavior. Drugs had been found in the American's room, and Bierer feared that this man might indeed be influencing other patients along paths detrimental to their mental health.

Following this part of the meeting, tea was served. The tea interlude is a regular ritual, obviously looked forward to and enjoyed by even the most withdrawn and regressed patients. There was a great deal of social chit-chat among the group members and several, including the social workers, made obvious efforts to involve the more reticent members in conversation. One of the patients introduced to me by Bierer spent most of the tea interval describing her experience with the club, and how it had rescued her from a life of disillusionment and loneliness and restored her mental health. The patients were apparently accustomed to giving testimonials of this kind, and did so quite readily.

Following the break for tea, the meeting resumed only to conduct some business regarding further plans of the group for an outing or activity of some sort, and then the meeting was adjourned. Many of the patients filed out in pairs or small groups actively engaged in animated conversation. A few drifted out the door in solitary silence. It seemed to me that the club meeting had been for these patients the brightest hours of their otherwise drab and lonely week.

12

Three unique programs

THE TAVISTOCK CENTRE

Familiarly referred to as "The Tavi," the Tavistock Clinic and the Tavistock Institute of Human Relations represent outstanding pillars in the psychiatric and psychoanalytic communities of Britain. Although many American psychiatrists are aware of the reputation of this famous institution, most are unfamiliar with its organization and unaware of the remarkable scope of its activities.

The Tavistock Clinic received its name from its earliest location in Tavistock Square, London, where it was founded in 1920 as one of the earliest psychiatric outpatient clinics in Britain. Although the clinic has changed its location several times, it has retained the original designation. From the first it had a psychodynamic orientation, established by its founding medical director, Dr. Hugh Crichton-Miller, an orientation which continues to the present day. The clinic moved to larger quarters in Malet Place, London, in 1932, and Dr. J. R. Rees became its second medical director in 1934. As the clinic continued to grow, its activities were expanded to include many educational and research endeavors. Over the next decade it became a leader in the teaching as well as the practice of dynamic psychiatry and psychology.

During World War II, many members of the clinic staff, including Dr. Rees, joined the armed forces, where they worked as a team on numer-

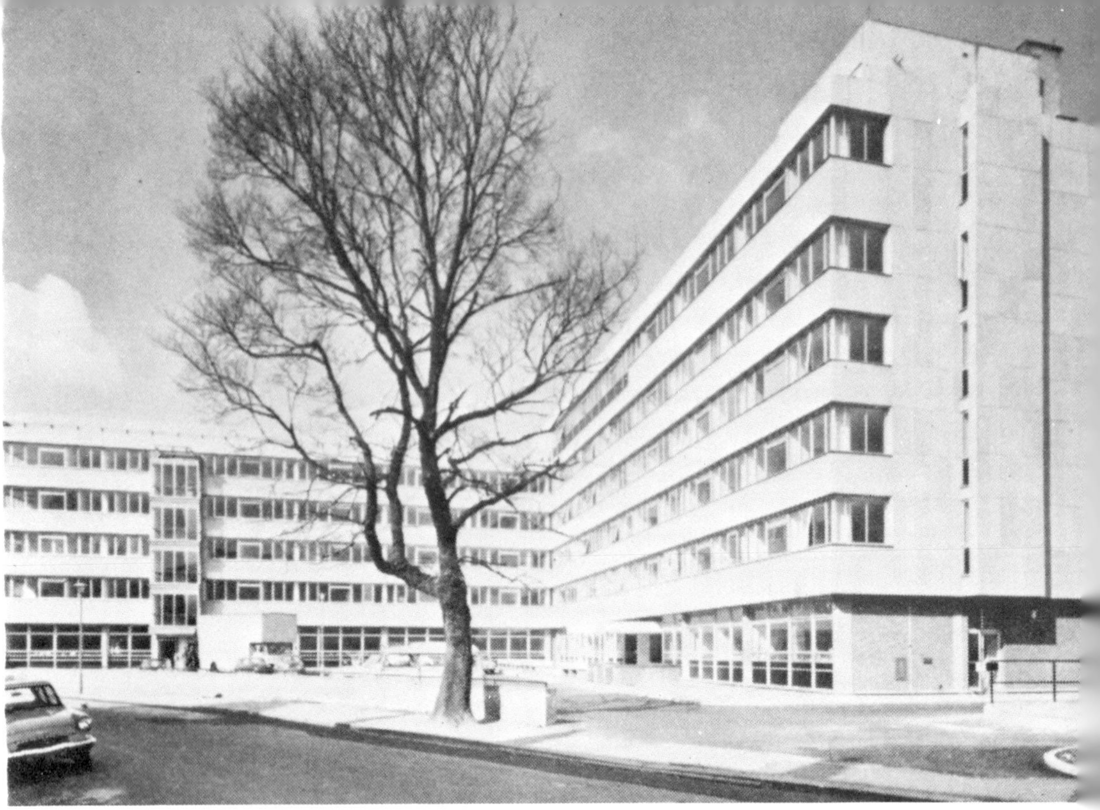

Tavistock Centre, London. (*Courtesy of C. Murray Parkes, M.D.*)

ous problems of morale, leadership, resocialization, the mentality of the enemy, management of the neurotic in military units, etc. As a result of these efforts, an interdisciplinary staff, sophisticated in the research methodologies of social psychology, was developed.

By the end of the war the clinic had moved to larger quarters in Beaumont Street, where the staff members returning from military service, together with many new staff members, established a new organization, the Tavistock Institute of Human Relations. The object of this sister organization, created with the help of Rockefeller Foundation support, was to continue and to extend the work developed by the staff's wartime experiences. The interdisciplinary efforts of the medically, socially, and psychoanalytically oriented institute staff were to be applied to studies of human resources and social organizations in group and institutional settings outside the medical field.

The Tavistock Clinic

The Tavistock Clinic became a part of the National Health Service in 1948. The Institute, however, remained as an independent body, free to pursue its own objectives but requiring its own sources of support.

By 1967 both the clinic and institute moved to a new large building constructed by the Ministry of Health on Belsize Lane, a quiet, tree-lined street in Hampstead, a pleasant residential area in northwest London. The modern building, known as the Tavistock Centre, provides adequate office space, classrooms, a staff cafeteria-lounge, and a fine library for both the clinic and the institute, many of whose staff members hold joint appointments. In addition, part of the building is occupied by the Child Guidance Training Centre, who also share the library and other facilities.

The primary role of the Tavistock Clinic is to provide treatment, hence its National Health Service support. It is administratively responsible to the St. Charles Group Hospital Management Committee. Internally, policy and planning for the clinic is the responsibility of a professional committee representative of its various clinical departments and professional disciplines. The clinic comprises an Adult Department, an Adolescent Department, and a Department of Children and Parents. It offers outpatient diagnostic and treatment services, as well as consultation. It is not responsible for a given catchment area and still provides service for many patients who first went into treatment when the clinic was at one of its earlier locations.

The Tavistock Institute of Human Relations

The Tavistock Institute of Human Relations is supported by grants from various foundations, student fees, and contracts to conduct particular investigations. Although education is one of its major activities, it is not connected with any university or medical school. The Institute is governed by a council, although its activities have been organized into five relatively autonomous units, each with its own subcouncil. These include: the School of Family Psychiatry and Community Mental Health; the Institute of Marital Studies; the Human Resources Centre; the Centre for Applied Social Research; and the Institute for Operational Research. The professional staff of approximately 65 represents a wide variety of disciplines, including over a dozen psychiatrists and psychoanalysts, most of whom are to be found at the School of Family Psychiatry.

The School of Family Psychiatry and Community Mental Health

The School of Family Psychiatry and Community Mental Health, organized as a postgraduate school, offers courses jointly with the Tavistock Clinic and the Institute of Marital Studies. It also has links with local authority and voluntary services. The objectives of the school include research, development of relevant theory, design of preventive and therapeutic services, and training of medical and non-medical, specialist and non-specialist personnel. Research activities have included inquiries into personality development, family function, diagnostic procedures, and therapeutic techniques. In the educational sphere a full range of training courses in family psychiatry and community mental health is offered to professionals representing the various mental health disciplines. The school offers intensive postgraduate training, including clinical work under supervision, via full-time, so-called "main" courses. In addition a range of day, evening, and short courses for professional groups is provided, including an annual four-day, summer seminar on the Public Health Aspects of Prevention led by Dr. Gerald Caplan of Harvard Medical School.

Nine full-time courses are offered by the School of Family Psychiatry and Community Mental Health. Three of these courses are specifically for psychiatrists, three for social workers, two for psychologists, and one for non-medical child psychotherapists. The latter program is probably the least familiar to American psychiatrists and will therefore be described below.

Between 1962 and 1968, 124 professional workers completed the full-time courses. Of these, 63 came from the field of social work, 32 from clinical or educational psychology, 19 from psychiatry, and 10 were child psychotherapists. This distribution of professional backgrounds may suggest a reason why "The Tavi" is the darling of the social work community of Britain.

THE CHILD PSYCHOTHERAPY TRAINING PROGRAM (NON-MEDICAL). The Child Psychotherapy Training Program in the Tavistock is one of three training programs approved by a recently formed Association of Child Psychotherapists and is the only one supported in part by the National Health Service. One of the programs is quite small. The other major program is located at the Hampstead Clinic, a few blocks away from the Tavistock, and is operated by Miss Anna Freud. It is probably the largest training program for child psychotherapists in the country. The program at the Hampstead Clinic is largely subsidized by grants from private foundations. The students are for the most part American and are supported by individual grants from the United States.

The program at the Tavistock, which is under the direction of Mrs. Martha Harris, used to be considerably smaller than the one at the Hampstead Clinic, but in recent years it has grown considerably. At the time of my visit, there were 18 clinical students and also 18 pre-clinical students. Of the 18 pre-clinicals, it was anticipated that probably 10 or 12 will go on to complete their clinical training. The growth can be appreciated when it is realized that there were only 10 graduates of the program in the previous six years.

The candidates for training in child psychotherapy must have a university background with honors, most usually in clinical psychology, but candidates also may have degrees in education, social work, etc. The review of the credentials of the applicants is most stringent, and selection depends upon the qualifications of the individuals. Candidates used to be selected on an *a priori* basis, but currently qualified applicants tend to be appointed to the pre-clinical part of the program during which time they are observed, their work with children is evaluated, and the selection proper for clinical training is made at the time the student completes his pre-clinical work.

All candidates must have a personal analysis with a member or associate member of the Institute of Psychoanalysis and are advised as to choice of analyst by the tutors responsible for the course. A number of candidates are already in personal analysis at the time that they come to the Child Psychotherapy Program. Others begin their analysis simultaneously with the beginning of their child psychotherapy training. The Tavistock will assist and advise the candidate on the choice of analyst, but if the candidate is already in analysis with someone, it is rare for the Tavistock to recommend change. However, it is not unusual for further personal analysis to be suggested.

All candidates for child psychotherapy training must at the time of enrollment as associate (pre-clinical) students be employed in some capacity in work with children. One or two years are required to complete the course of work for associate students. During this time the candidate attends a well organized program of seminars including one wherein they discuss their own work with children in the setting in which they are then currently employed. In this way the staff of the program become acquainted with the kind of work the student is doing and is capable of. During the first year, the candidates attend common lectures, seminars, and other courses shared by all full-time students at the Tavistock, whatever their professional discipline or particular course of study.

Child psychotherapy students are not permitted to take on supervisory cases until they have completed at least one year of personal analysis. At that time they will be assigned a case, and over a period of time, three cases, consisting of one child under five, one between five and eleven years old, and one adolescent, each to be seen for five-times-a-week psychoanalytic treatment. Each case is supervised by a psychoanalyst; the first two supervisors generally are on the staff of the Tavistock, while the third supervisor may be on the staff or may be an outside psychoanalyst. In addition to the three intensive analytic cases, the child psychotherapist sees a number of children in other kinds of therapeutic relationships, such as once-a-week psychotherapy. They also work with parents and families of children. Part of the program includes visits to homes for the purpose of observing child development at first hand. In this respect the child psychotherapy program at the Tavistock differs from that at the Hampstead Clinic, where almost all of the emphasis is placed upon working with children in five-days-per-week psychoanalysis. Thus the people Miss Freud is training are really lay child-psychoanalysts, rather than child psychotherapists in the stricter sense.

This difference of emphasis coincides with the difference in clinical approach of the two institutions. While the orientation of the Tavistock is psychoanalytic, the clinical work with children is not conducted along traditionally psychoanalytic lines. Rather, psychoanalytic knowledge is used for understanding the problem, while the therapeutic approach is more eclectic.

While the staff of the Tavistock Centre are subsidized by the National Health Service, which is thereby subsidizing the Child Psychotherapy Program, there are no direct grants to the program *per se*. Nor are there any grants for the child psychotherapy students at the Tavistock. Thus, considering the time involved, the payment of fees for their course work, and the cost for the personal analysis, it is rather expensive for a candidate to undertake child psychotherapy training. Since the remuneration afterwards is no greater than it would be for the ordinary clinical psychologist, the child psychotherapy students are quite serious, and their motivation is very high.

The child psychotherapy training program lasts three to four years, following which the graduate becomes eligible for membership in the Society of Child Psychotherapists and generally obtains employment in a school for disturbed children, a child guidance clinic, or a hospital outpatient department. Usually, patients begun in treatment at the Tavistock Clinic by child psychotherapy candidates continue in treatment with the therapist after graduation, since psychotherapy, and particularly child analysis, may go on for a number of years before termination.

While there are some members of the British Psychoanalytic Institute who look askance at the child psychotherapy program, most analysts regard it quite favorably, and it has a generally good reputation.

COMMUNITY CONSULTATION—ST. CHRISTOPHER'S HOSPICE. A major goal of the School of Family Psychiatry and Community Mental Health is to foster working relationships between psychiatrists and other helping professions. Toward this end, the school offers consultative services to various agencies for mental health problems encountered during the course of the agency's usual activities. Such community consultations usually include some inservice training. Most of these activities are conducted in collaboration with the staff of the Institute of Marital Studies and/or the Tavistock Clinic.

Community consultations are provided on a regular basis to schools, including a College of Education, borstals and training schools, a probation hostel for girls, the YWCA, Family Planning Association, the

Richmond Fellowship, and similar agencies. A rather unusual recipient of the consultation service is the St. Christopher's Hospice, Sydenham, a hospital for terminally ill patients.

The consultant to St. Christopher's is Dr. C. Murray Parkes, who works full-time at the Tavistock. He makes weekly visits to the hospice, seeing patients who have psychiatric problems and discussing their management with the nursing staff. He also meets with a medical social worker, called an almoner. Most of his work, however, is directly with the patients themselves. Dr. Parkes is uniquely suited for his consultant role. He has had a long interest in the problems of bereavement and reactions to loss. In addition to conducting research in this area over a period of years, he worked regularly with the residents and officials of Aberfan, Wales, for 18 months, following the devastating mine disaster of 1967.

St. Christopher's Hospice is a religious and medical foundation caring for "those in pain and suffering due to advanced cancer and other long-term illness." Opened in 1967, the hospice is operated as a voluntary institution but maintains links with the National Health Service, so that most patients can obtain care without charge. It is housed in a relatively new and quite modern building, especially constructed for the purpose. There are 54 beds in the main wing, chiefly for terminal cancer patients, and an adjacent structure, called the Draper's Wing, provides bed-sitter accommodations for 16 aged and infirm individuals (108). The patient areas of the main wing are well designed and are constructed in units of three groups of four patients each. An area for visitors runs along one side of the patient area, while a corridor for nursing activities runs down the opposite side. The rooms are light, airy, and cheerful, although essentially functional.

About 90% of the patients admitted die in the hospice; 10% are discharged to other hospitals or nursing homes, or return home. A recently developed outpatient program and Family Service Project has enabled the hospice to care for an additional 70 patients in their own homes, although many of them make several trips back and forth to the hospice for brief inpatient stays.* Almost one-half of the patients die within two weeks of hospitalization, an additional one-third die within two months, and 18% remain over two months. The hospice is ideally suited to cope with the intense dependency of the short-stay patients. For those with longer survivals, there is the problem of maintaining autonomy in the face of extreme feelings of helplessness. For the increasing number of patients who die in their homes, the nurses of the hospice provide extra support to the family doctors and district nurses.

*Personal communication to the author from Cicely Saunders, M.D., April 6, 1973.

The hospice is well staffed, having a nurse to patient ratio of 1.25 to 1. In part, the ability to maintain this staffing pattern is due to the establishment of a nursery and playroom to provide day-care for the children of married nurses; this enables their mothers to work at the hospice. In addition to the regular staff, there are approximately 100 volunteers from the local community who participate in every department of the hospice (108).

St. Christopher's Hospice was founded by its current director, Dr. Cicely Saunders, who is indeed a most remarkable person. She had a background in nursing and social work before taking medical training. Of all the institutions I visited, this was one of only two where the original founder was still active, and it was immediately obvious that her presence at the hospice was a major factor in the institution's success. Dr. Saunders has great charm and charisma and a gift for inspiring the staff and setting a model of religious dedication for others to emulate. Her continuing presence is also noted in the maintenance of financial support for the hospice, which is a reflection of the successful investment of her energies in fund-raising. While approximately two-thirds of St. Christopher's financial needs are provided through its links with the National Health Service, the remainder must be obtained annually through contributions from charitable foundations and individual gifts.

Although patients are admitted on a non-denominational basis, the hospice maintains its own chapel and chaplain. Most of the staff are imbued with a religious dedication towards easing the final hours of suffering of terminally ill patients. There is no Bible-quoting or evangelism, merely a spiritual conviction that they are doing God's work. The staff are well prepared to cope with death and dying and are quite expert in handling patients' questions about their condition, how long they have to live, etc. In addition, staff members are exceptionally skillful at working with the families of patients, both in preparing for and reacting to the death of a loved one. Death occurs with dignity and decorum, and the families are treated with respect. Despite the fact that most cases end in death, the mood and atmosphere are far from depressing. It is, in fact, a surprisingly bright, even cheerful place.

Visiting is encouraged. There are no regular visiting hours; visitors may come at any time and remain as long as they like. A special room for visitors is provided where they may sit apart from the patients, or they may remain with the patients as they wish.

Patients are cared for in a very loving and considerate way, but every effort is made to activate them as much as possible. Patients are moved about in their beds rather than via cart or wheelchair. When a patient is admitted he is moved directly from his ambulance to his bed, which is then taken to the ward. When a patient dies, his bed is removed and taken by a special elevator to the morgue.

Drugs are used quite liberally, particularly heroin and morphine in the so-called "Brompton Mixture," consisting of morphine or diamorphine (heroin) (at present the preferred drug of Dr. Saunders), plus small amounts of cocaine in gin or some other form of alcohol. Some doctors add honey or other sweetening, and others include syrup of chlorpromazine or prochlorperazine. This mixture has the effect not only of easing pain, but of making the patient "a great deal happier." The management of pain by routine administration of drugs prevents psychological dependence. Patients are free of pain and do not have to ask continually for relief. There is no concern that these patients will become physiologically addicted or drug dependent, since most are close to death anyway.

Various combinations of drugs are used for each patient until pain is controlled and discomfort eased. The Department of Clinical Studies is conducting an active research program on the comparative effectiveness of the various preparations in easing pain. This study is unusual in that in addition to the direct analgesic action of the drugs, it also takes into account the effect of the therapeutic environment of the ward in easing the suffering of patients. In addition to the use of drugs, the hospice retains the services of a consultant anesthesiologist who, in selected cases, does spinal nerve blocks for pain relief.

At times the psychiatric problem about which Dr. Parkes consults is one of depression, but not nearly so frequently as one might suppose in a hospital of this type. Parkes is concerned with the problems that arise as the patient and his family struggle with the realities of coming to terms with dying. Another sphere in which Parkes functions relates to his interest in bereavement. The Family Service Project, which he directs, attempts to establish relationships with the families of patients who have died in the hospice, who may be unable to cope with their grief and the stresses of life caused by their loss. While at first reluctant to intrude upon the grieving family, Parkes had merely made the service "available" to anyone who cared to use it. He informs me that since 1970, however, the approach to the family has been more direct, and there has been a gratifying acceptance of the support and counsel offered by this program.

To sum up this remarkable institution: the quality of care generally is unusually high, the dedication of the staff is exceptional, and the tone of the institution probably could not be maintained without the religious structure.

YOUNG PEOPLES COUNSELLING SERVICE. A more service-oriented activity of the School of Family Psychiatry and Community

Mental Health is the Young Peoples Counselling Service (YPCS), which works in close collaboration with the Adolescent Department of the Tavistock Clinic. This program is essentially a diagnostic and brief psychotherapy service to help young people deal with the kinds of problems they themselves present. It does not provide long-term treatment. In many instances it serves as a referral service, putting the young people in touch with other agencies better suited to help them with their particular problems.

The Young Peoples Counselling Service is an interdisciplinary effort which has successfully provided a needed service over several years and has served as a model for others. In 1959 a group of distinguished citizens, concerned with problems of delinquency and troubled by the fact that young people were unable to receive professional help until a major crisis had occurred, decided to develop a consulting service so that help would be available earlier, and hopefully major difficulties could be avoided. After two years of planning, and with the help of financial support from the van Leer Foundation, a private philanthropic fund, the service was opened in June 1961, as a walk-in service for 15-21 year olds, offering consultation to clients for all sorts of problems. The emphasis was on brief intervention and help with problem-solving, using the strengths of the young people. The YPCS was intended to be a professional service, available when most needed, although the service was inaugurated on only a part-time basis. Other goals were to do research, to carry out educational programs, and to issue publications.

The YPCS staff first opened their doors in space made available by the Hampstead Borough Council. To attract clients, they have advertised both directly in the newspapers and indirectly since 1965. In addition to the psychologists and social workers making up the original professional staff, the YPCS added a consultant psychiatrist, and also a general practitioner as a medical advisor for physical problems. However, their intention was to soft-pedal the medical aspects of the agency. The medical specialists saw their clients in their own consulting rooms rather than at the Young Peoples Centre in order to avoid a psychiatric or medical identification for the service. The physicians also provided consultations to the staff of the Young Peoples Counselling Service.

The group later obtained its own quarters at Swiss Cottage. Psychoanalysts were added to the staff, thereby enriching the depth and scope of services already provided by the psychiatric social workers and psychologists. The service continued to function with a part-time professional staff on a part-time basis, open three evenings a week plus Saturday morning. The YPCS. had two full-time secretaries and two part-time receptionists. The service was so successful that a short time later a branch office was opened at Nottinghill Gate.

The YPCS set up a field work training program, which was handled by professional subcommittees. They ran courses for people working with adolescents and young adults, and became a very closely knit team. The van Leer Foundation increased its support by £2,000 a year in order to provide psychotherapy for those who needed it. More recently, however, the van Leer Foundation withdrew its support for consulting services, although it agreed to continue its support for research. As a consequence, the group closed its Nottinghill Gate branch, and then its Swiss Cottage office as well, and moved to the Tavistock. At the time of my visit, a review was underway of 100 cases seen at the Tavistock during 1968.

A number of other groups have taken note of their work and have sought to emulate them. Some of these voluntary community groups, others are in hospitals, still others are in local authorities. These people often have come for guidance in setting up their own programs. However, in practice the programs supposedly modelled on the YPCS vary a great deal, employing both nonprofessional and professional workers, both paid and voluntary.

Their present program is "no longer so ambitious or pioneering," according to Mr. F. H. G. Balfour, a psychologist who joined the service when it came to the Tavistock, and who since was named chairman of the group. "However, the problems are the same as in the pre-Tavistock days." Their present focus is mainly on service, although they continue to do some education and research. The training offered is mostly for internal Tavistock students in clinical psychology and case work, but they hope to extend this to extramural teaching.

Clients continue to increase in number each year, showing that the service continues to fill a recognized need. Each time there is a newspaper article on the function of the service, there is a deluge of clients, confirming that the total need is not yet being tapped.

The brief nature of the contact is spelled out to the client when he first arrives, although he is generally not told the professional identity of the person he sees. The service seems most appropriate to those in the 17-21 age range who are not sick enough to require psychiatric treatment.

The YPCS team originally conceived of their activities as a drop-in service, but in practice this has not been their primary mode of operation, nor do they now consider themselves in this light, although they still have occasional drop-ins, anyway. Most clients call for appointments in advance and are willing to wait a few days to be seen. The present staff consists of members of the Tavistock Clinic's Adolescent Department, who work part-time with the YPCS. There are no emergency services, but as has been noted, they will see the occasional drop-in.

The time given to the clients is not in the amounts typical for psychotherapy, but is rather the more limited kind of counsel that one might expect from a general practitioner or a teacher. A psychoanalytical orientation is maintained, however, and they believe they have demonstrated a correlation between the dynamic nature of the initial psychiatric interview and the success of the brief intervention offered. Nevertheless, they have not yet been able to determine why it is they may succeed or fail with any given case. Balfour suggests, "Perhaps it is just that some of the clients are very responsive to brief help and/or some professionals are very good at doing it." In fact, they have no follow-up whatsoever and frequently are ignorant of whether or not their efforts have indeed been successful.

There is a growing concern about becoming swamped by cases. The idea of the YPCS is to help the client use his life more efficiently and effectively, and they are trying to learn more about whom they can help most and whose problems are not suited for their service. According to Balfour, "It is tempting to be omnipotent and to manage the patient, but this temptation must be resisted."

Twenty-eight percent of YPCS clients are self-referred, 20% are referred by social workers, 17% by friends and relatives, 14% by parents, 14% by schools and 7% by the general practitioners. There is roughly an equal number of males and females. Complaints are mostly interpersonal or intra-psychic difficulties, such as depressions, problems with the boyfriend or girlfriend, school problems, employment problems, complaints of anxiety, drug-taking problems, disagreements with parents, etc. Forty percent of clients have lost either one or both parents through death or divorce.

Part of the YPCS activity is a screening function. Thirty percent of the people coming to them are subsequently referred to other agencies. Thirty-nine percent of the contacts are terminated by mutual consent, which is generally regarded by the group as indicating a successful outcome. There is no other follow-up to measure success. Eighteen percent have an unsatisfactory termination. Thirty-one percent of clients have only one interview, 19% have two interviews, and another 25% have five or more interviews.

The present intake of the YPCS is 220 cases per year. Those under 17 years of age make up 21% of the case load, and those over 22 make up 15%; the vast majority, 64%, are between the ages of 17 and 21. In treating each case, therapists aim to select the most prominent problem nearest to the surface for their focus, limiting their efforts to this problem and emphasizing to the client that he can return later for further help.

RESEARCH PROJECTS. The School of Family Psychiatry and Community Mental Health maintains an active program of research, with emphasis upon studies of personality development, family interrelationships, diagnostic procedures for assessing personality and family functioning, and therapeutic techniques. Several projects describe and record the behavior of children, adults, and families in different settings over periods of time lasting from a few months to a year or two. A period is selected either because it is known to be a phrase of rapid personality change, such as the first year of life or puberty, or because the subject is being exposed to a major change in his life space; for example, the separation of child from mother, loss of husband by wife, amputation of limb, or transition from school to college.

Studies of how the young child responds during and after periods of separation from his mother have long been among the central research issues at the Tavistock. Dr. John Bowlby, who has been working on these problems for some years, is preparing a comprehensive work entitled *Attachment and Loss,* to appear in three volumes, of which two have been published: *Attachment* (1969) and *Separation, Anxiety and Anger* (1973) (London: Hogarth Press and Institute for Psycho-Analysis; New York: Basic Books).

In a related area, Mr. and Mrs. J. Robertson have been working on the preparation of film and written publications deriving from their ongoing project, a study of young children in brief separation. They are also working on two other projects, one on day nurseries and the other on the care of young children in long-stay hospitals.

Dr. Dorothy Heard has continued to work on the interactive behavior of young children, supported by a grant from the Northwestern Metropolitan Regional Hospital Board. She is also undertaking a pilot project to study the effect on a marriage of the advent of the first baby.

Related projects, stimulated by the Tavistock studies in this field, have been developed at other centers as well. Two with which Dr. Bowlby has especially close links are those of Professor Mary Salter Ainsworth at Johns Hopkins, and of Professor Robert Hinde in Cambridge. Professor Ainsworth, who worked with Dr. Bowlby and Mr. Robertson at the Tavistock during 1950-54, is engaged in developmental studies of human infants and mothers. Professor Hinde, a member of the school's sub-council, is making comparable studies of monkey infants and mothers.

Reaction to loss in adult life is also a major research interest. Dr. Parkes is engaged in a number of projects in this area. Drawing on his experience of over ten years' work in this field, he has completed a book entitled *Studies in Grief in Adult Life* (New York: International Universities Press, 1973) that describes the principal findings of recent work and some of the implications it has for helping the bereaved. Parkes is also engaged in a study of the reaction to amputation of a limb and is directing a cooperative Anglo-American project in which widows and widowers are being studied during their first four years of bereavement and compared with a control group of married subjects. These studies are in addition to those already mentioned on terminal cancer at St. Christopher's Hospice, Sydenham.

At present almost all the research undertaken at the School of Family Psychiatry and Community Mental Health is supported by *ad hoc* grants obtained by the research workers themselves. The role of the school is to identify promising individuals and lines of work, to aid them in obtaining grants, and to provide them with administrative and library facilities and the necessary space. It is presently seeking additional money to encourage promising work to the point at which it can obtain funds elsewhere and also to provide for overhead expenses.

The Institute of Marital Studies

The Institute of Marital Studies (IMS), formerly the Family Discussion Bureau, acquired its present name in late 1968. It first began in 1948 as an experimental unit of the Family Welfare Association, specializing in marital and family problems. Over the years the IMS developed a close working relationship with the Tavistock Clinic and the Tavistock Institute of Human Relations, finally becoming a part of the institute in 1956. Here it has continued to work closely with the staffs of the clinic and other units of the institute.

The activities of the IMS encompass service, training, and research. Service chiefly consists of social casework with couples experiencing marital problems. The caseworkers of the IMS treat a considerable number of couples referred by physicians and social agencies or who are self-referred, and the case load continues to increase.

Training activities range over a wide area, from casework seminars offered at the Institute for Marital Studies to advanced courses for supervisors and senior caseworkers given as far afield as Haifa, Israel, and the Smith College School of Social Work in the United States. The IMS participates on a collaborative basis in many of the courses offered by the School of Family Psychiatry and Community Mental Health. All told, they teach over 600 case workers and allied professionals each year.

Research has centered chiefly on the causes of marital disturbances. The IMS recently distilled 20 years of investigation into the causes of divorce into a document which was submitted to the Parliament in connection with its consideration of changes in the divorce laws. The IMS staff have also studied the forces favoring cohesiveness in marriage and the effectiveness of casework intervention in troubled marriages.

The Human Resources Centre

The Human Resources Centre has engaged in numerous, highly diverse research activities. Investigations include surveys of career expectations of graduates and school-leavers, studies of dual-career families, surveys of administrative managers, the life styles and work systems of seamen, the design of a rubber fabrication factory, problems of work roles in a steel-making plant, and studies of the relationship between stress and performance. Many investigations are undertaken under contract with industrial firms, government agencies, and private foundations. The staff also publish a journal called *Human Relations* and have presented lectures or engaged in collaborative educational and research ventures at various centers in many parts of the world.

The Centre for Applied Social Research

The Centre for Applied Social Research conducts studies on a wide range of social issues. Subjects of investigation have included social policy, the transition from school to work, poverty, residential institutions for the physically handicapped and chronically ill, approved schools (i.e., reformatories), relationships between mental hospitals and local communities, sociological factors relating to home ownership, industrial productivity, and organizational systems. Most of these investigations have been sponsored by various governmental departments. In addition, consultative services are offered to a variety of institutions including banks, industrial firms, publishing houses, church organizations, etc.

Training is another major activity of the Centre. They offer short courses, conduct study groups, and hold residential conferences both at the Tavistock Centre and at other institutes throughout Britain and in other countries.

The Institute for Operational Research

The Institute for Operational Research seeks to apply its area of specialization to all levels of decision-making, from day-to-day management through planning and the formation of strategic policy. These have been focused in recent years chiefly on the hospital services, public planning, and certain industrial situations.

Its staff have been working with the hospital authorities on a variety of problems under the sponsorship of the Ministry of Health ever since January 1968. Projects have included the development of the operational policies for new hospitals, coordinating information about patients and hospital activities, and studies of length of hospital stay and cost effectiveness. In the area of public planning, the institute has made a study of the operations of the city of Coventry, analyzing the governmental decision-making processes. This study, supported by the Nuffield Foundation, has been published as a book, *Local Government and Strategic Choice.* They have also been working on a study of multiorganizational problems under the sponsorship of the Social Science Research Council.

The industrial program includes a project "Aids to Decision Making and Design" supported by the Science Research Council. They have worked on several problems in the building industry, including a commission by the National Board for Prices and Incomes to study wage structure and productivity in the construction industry. A number of manpower studies have been carried out under various auspices, and members of the staff have served as consultants to a variety of industrial and other organizations.

THE INSTITUTE OF FAMILY PSYCHIATRY

The Institute of Family Psychiatry is a specialized service, unique in the United Kingdom, located in Ipswich, Suffolk. It was established in 1949 by Dr. John G. Howells, who remains its present director. The Institute is an experimental unit for teaching and research in family psychiatry which is part of the Ipswich Hospital, a large general hospital. It serves a catchment area of approximately 300,000 people who reside in the city and surrounding rural areas.

The unit is housed in a separate three-story building adjoining the general hospital complex. It is situated amid pleasant surroundings at the top of a steep hill. Across the street is a large public park. The unit encloses a sheltered courtyard which contains an attractive garden and a number of rabbit hutches. On the ground floor, adjoining the garden, is a waiting room. Usually the adults use the waiting room, while the children wait in the garden. Also on the ground floor are a general clerical office, an occupational therapy office, and three playrooms used for child psychotherapy. In addition, there are a clinical examining room and a kitchen used for preparing tea. On the floor above is a suite of four rooms occupied by the social work staff, a staff library, and four psychiatrists' offices. There is also a large office for the director. The top floor houses three clinical psychology offices and a room for the research assistant.

Although the building is old, it has been kept up well and considerable attention has been paid to the decor. The furnishings, color scheme, and general ambience service to create a warm, relaxed atmosphere.

The staff consists of three psychiatrists (including Dr. Howells, the director of the institute), three clinical psychologists, four occupational therapists, an art therapist, four social workers, a research assistant, and a clerical staff of six people. In addition, there is a receptionist and a porter.

The present clinical program evolved over the years beginning as a child psychiatry program in 1949. Since it is impossible to provide psychi-

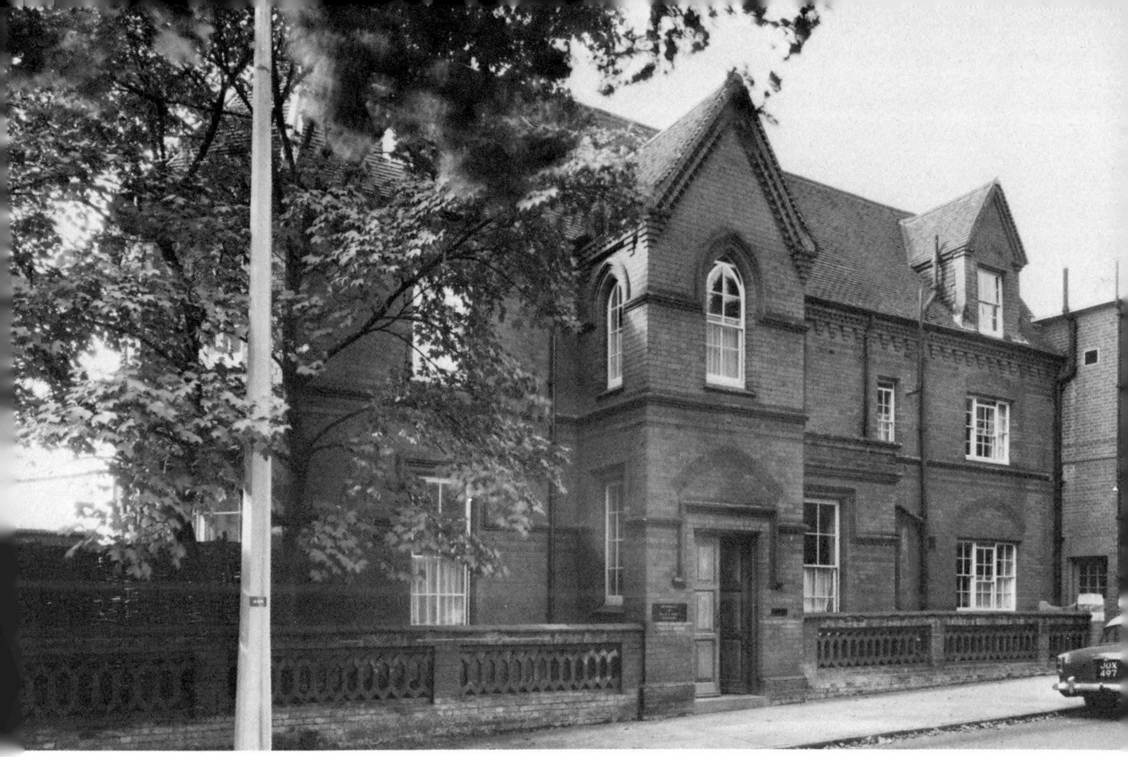

The Institute of Family Psychiatry, Ipswich. (*Courtesy of John Howells, M.D.*)

atric services to children without also involving the parents, the adult family members were brought into treatment quite early (68). It soon developed that many families had several children who needed help, and this was next offered to all children in the family. Soon an adolescent clinic was added, and by 1957, another clinic, specifically for dealing with marital problems, was opened. Thus by this time, the department was already dealing with entire families and was renamed the Department of Child and Family Psychiatry. As Howells further developed his approach to bring the primary focus of treatment upon the family as a unit, the role of the child as patient was de-emphasized, and the name of the department was again changed to the Department of Family Psychiatry. The department achieved Institute status in 1967.

The clinical approach developed by Howells is generally well known in the United States, for he has written extensively on the subject and has made many lecture tours in this country. In particular, Howells' book, *Theory and Practice of Family Psychiatry,* describes both his theoretical ideas and clinical approach (66).

According to Howells, a sick individual is a sign of a sick family.

Thus in his approach, the entire family unit, rather than a particular designated family member, becomes the patient. No matter which individual may be referred by the general practitioner or social agency, the entire family is quickly brought into treatment at the institute. Services offered include evaluation, often via "family group diagnosis," a term used by Howells to mean that all members of the household are interviewed together, including nannies and lodgers who may play a role in the family dynamics at the time. The diagnostic interview may be supplemented by the use of the "Family Relations Indicator" (70), an innovation devised at the Institute for the exploration of family relationships.

The major therapeutic approaches employed include family psychotherapy, and "vector therapy." The latter term was coined by Howells to indicate efforts aimed at rebalancing the field of forces impinging upon the family from within or without.

Howells sees society as a vast field of forces in which the elements–i.e., culture, community, neighborhood, family, and individual–each have equal significance. Imbalance of the emotional forces between the elements can bring harm, while they can be repatterned to promote well-being. The ultimate goal of vector therapy is a "reshaping over the generations of the emotional strata of society." This requires an extensive study of social organizations, institutions, roles, standards, and aims in order to achieve the ultimate goal–what Howells calls "the salutiferous society."

In addition to its extensive clinical responsibilities, the institute maintains a number of active educational programs, a rather remarkable achievement when one considers that it has neither university nor medical school affiliation. These programs include a two-year postgraduate course for training occupational therapists in play diagnosis and play therapy, a year-round generic course in family psychiatry for members of all the helping professions, weekly sessions for general practitioners, and special week-long courses offered annually to particular professional groups, including nurses, social workers, psychologists, and physicians, including psychiatrists. In addition, it maintains an active inservice training program for its own staff.

There is also a research program, one aspect of which has focused upon clinical problems, such as studies in family group diagnosis, family group therapy, vector therapy, and the Family Relations Indicator. The institute also operates a special experimental adolescent unit run on family lines. The other emphasis of the research effort has been on the systematic study of the psychopathology of problem families, an investigation of the effects of separation upon children, and a study of patterns of family member interaction designated the "Thousand Family Study."

THE INSTITUTE OF PSYCHIATRY AND MAUDSLEY HOSPITAL, LONDON

The most important facility in Britain for the teaching of postgraduate psychiatry is the University of London Institute of Psychiatry, where Professor Sir Denis Hill is head of the Department of Psychiatry. The institute is associated with the Maudsley and Bethlem Royal Hospitals. Its varied program includes research and public health work in addition to clinical training in psychiatry, and it also serves as an important training center for nurses, occupational therapists, psychologists, and social workers. Apart from psychiatry, there are departments of biochemistry, biometrics, neurophysiology, neuropathology, and psychology. Within the department of psychiatry there are chairs of epidemiology, social psychiatry, and forensic psychiatry. The institute's outstanding staff of teachers and researchers have a high reputation, and it is considered a distinct honor to be offered a staff appointment. A substantial proportion of the psychiatric educators of Britain took their training there.

Maudsley was organized in the twenties, and in 1948, as a consequence of the reorganization of services under the National Health Service Act, the Bethlem Royal Hospital (once "Bedlam") was added to it. Maudsley is located in a lower-middle-class and working-class area of southeast London called Camberwell. Across the street (Denmark Hill) is Kings College Hospital, an undergraduate teaching hospital (i.e., medical school) affiliated with the University of London. The main buildings of the Maudsley date from just before World War I and are now distinctly old-fashioned. A new, modern, purpose-built Institute of Psychiatry building was opened in 1967. It faces on de Crespigny Park, around the corner from Denmark Hill, and is connected by tunnels and other links to the other older buildings. The inpatient services include a Metabolic Unit, a Children's Department, an Adolescent Unit, and a Geriatric Unit; there are also facilities for neurophysiology and endocrinology. There are drug and alcohol addiction units, a unit for patients with epilepsy, and three inpatient psychotherapy units. The outpatient service is located in a more modern building, which, however, is no more impressive in its appearance than are its surrounding structures. Nearby is the Maudsley Day Hospital, occupying a rather run-down, converted four-story house.

Inpatient Facilities

The medical staff of the Maudsley and Bethlem Royal Hospitals also serve St. Francis Hospital which, in the past, served as a receiving hospital to which psychiatric emergencies from throughout London were admitted—a sort of British "Bellevue." This function was changed, however, when the Maudsley took responsibility to serve a catchment area in 1967.

Initially, the Maudsley, like other teaching hospitals, did not have responsibility for serving a particular catchment area. Admissions to teaching hospitals are typically based upon the teaching value of the case, and patients may be admitted even from remote parts of the country. However, many members of the staff felt that it would be advantageous to the research and teaching activities of the Maudsley to undertake responsibility for a catchment area. At the same time the area served would benefit greatly from the high caliber of the staff, facilities, and services offered by the Maudsley. For a number of years, therefore, the staff worked towards the development of a Maudsley catchment area in Camberwell. These arrangements were completed in 1967.

It was understood that, despite undertaking responsibility for providing comprehensive mental health service to the area, Maudsley would continue to accept patients from a much wider area in support of its other teaching and research activities; in fact, most of its beds will still be used in this way.

To provide service to its new catchment area, and at the same time continue its traditional "teaching hospital" caseload, a redeployment of its facilities was necessary. Therefore, in 1967, the St. Francis Hospital closed its doors for three months and underwent a significant reorganization.

Following its reopening, its 60 psychiatric beds were allocated for medium- and short-stay patients (up to 12 months). Of these, 45 beds were reserved for patients from the Camberwell catchment area, while the other 15 beds were to be used for patients from other parts of London. At the same time the Maudsley set aside 90 beds to accommodate patients from the Camberwell catchment area requiring both short-term and medium-term hospitalization. A few patients were still admitted to Cane Hill Hospital (a State Hospital some 15 miles away), particularly if suffering from dementia or in need of long-term care, but they remained under the care of Maudsley physicians. It is planned that these patients also will be treated within the district facilities by 1975. It was not possible to carry out this plan without difficulties, but the number of Camberwell patients admitted to Cane Hill has dropped dramatically, and the plan is so far running on schedule. An interesting development has been the reduction in the total number of beds occupied by schizophrenic patients as efforts have been made increasingly to treat them in day-hospital or outpatient settings within the community. On the other hand, there has been a temporary increase in the occupancy of hospital beds by patients with other diagnoses such as psychoneuroses, addictions, and sociopathic conditions. In the past the latter groups had not been hospitalized to any great extent, but once the beds had been vacated by the schizophrenics, an extra influx of this patient group into the hospital took place, though this has now levelled out.

The general emphasis on community mental health has had a beneficial effect upon the approaches to treatment of mental patients. For example, while St. Francis Hospital in the past offered no more than diagnosis and "disposal," it is now primarily a very active treatment center.

The Social Psychiatry Research Unit

When the Maudsley assumed responsibility for the Camberwell catchment area, one of its major objectives was the evaluation of the effectiveness of its community mental health approaches. This evaluative research is conducted at the Social Psychiatry Unit under the direction of Dr. John Wing. The Research Unit is housed in the modern Institute of Psychiatry building at the Maudsley but is supported by the Medical Research Council, a national agency set up to promote all forms of medical research. Dr. Wing divides his time between his research, clinical work, and teaching (he is professor of social psychiatry at the University of London Institute of Psychiatry and at the London School of Hygiene). Wing has been engaged in the study of the effectiveness of mental health services for the past 15 years and has published a great deal in this field (113, 114). As the emphasis on community mental health approaches developed in Britain, he and his group made studies of various efforts in this direction as they were carried out in different parts of England, specifically including London, Colchester, and Nottingham.

In 1965, Wing and his colleagues began establishing a psychiatric register and collecting data on psychiatric experiences with the population of Camberwell, which contains approximately 175,000 people and now comprises the Maudsley's catchment area. Wing now feels that, for research purposes, it would be valuable to have an even larger catchment area in order to collect enough cases of certain types which are more difficult to find.

The Camberwell Register

Dr. Lorna Wing supervises the Camberwell Psychiatric Register, of which Mrs. Anthea Hailey, a sociologist and statistician, is in day to day charge (115). In addition, the staff includes seven clerical people whose job it is to visit the various agencies serving psychiatric patients from the Camberwell area and review their records and charts in order to dig out the statistical information necessary to keep the register up to date. This is a full-time job and a rather difficult one, but they find it impossible to rely solely upon other agencies to complete the necessary forms. Therefore, this "digging out" must be done on a regular, ongoing basis.

The data which are collected in this manner, along with other more readily available data on the Camberwell patients, are fed into the computer at monthly intervals. Many technical problems are involved in maintaining the register, and it is necessary to employ a computer programmer almost full-time to handle the programming of the Camberwell data. The annual cost for maintaining the baseline data is £2,000. If statistical correlations, development of charts, or other analyses of the data are being performed, the cost runs to £6,000. The register is part of the Social Psychiatry Unit, and the Department of Health contributes towards its cost (115, 116).

The collected data are in the form of loose sheets of foolscap which are not in numerical order. The data are punched on paper tape and fed to a computer which supplies a print-out in numerical order. The print-out is next checked against the master data for errors, and transcribed onto magnetic tape. Two tapes are coded simultaneously, one as a master copy, the second as a duplicate, which is the working copy. The purpose of duplicate tapes is for protection in the event of damage to one of them Strict precautions are taken to preserve confidentiality.

In addition to the data recorded on the tapes, a master file card system is maintained at the Maudsley. At the time of my visit, there were something like 8,000 cards on file there. There is a card for each patient from the Camberwell area who has come into contact with a psychiatrist since 1964; every hospitalization, outpatient visit, and admission to day care or other facilities is noted. A specific length of tape is allotted to each patient, and provision made for recording subsequent data. Even with all of the efforts to elicit the material from the patient's chart, there are nevertheless problems in collecting and maintaining the data accurately and adequately.

I discussed with Dr. John Wing the findings based on the register, which relate to the effectiveness of the community mental health program. He said that initially there had been a tendency to think that community mental health programs would bring mentally ill patients into treatment very early, and that early intervention would result in the patients being cured before any chronic disabilities developed. Thus, an early hope was that within a period of time the mental hospitals could be abolished altogether. Studies have demonstrated that these expectations are not yet realized, because some mental illness is chronic in nature and generally not susceptible to "cure." It therefore requires a program for ongoing care in any event. While early intervention may make treatment approaches simpler and easier, it does not altogether avoid chronicity.

Wing studied in particular three community care programs, one very advanced, integrated, and comprehensive, the other two more traditional. The outcomes for schizophrenic patients and the problems of relatives were not, however, very different. On the other hand, when studying long-stay inpatients in the same three hospitals, he found clear evidence that "institutionalism" could be prevented by an active program. Other rehabilitation studies confirmed these results with long-stay patients. The increased attention given to patients and the vigor of the approaches of recent years does seem to have a more beneficial effect upon the patient population generally than the more traditional custodial approaches.

As a result of his studies, Wing now believes that the main emphasis of the community mental health approach should be on secondary and tertiary prevention rather than primary prevention. He feels that since mental illness is often chronic, the rehabilitative approach is probably the most effective way to benefit these patients. Primary prevention efforts are worthwhile, but they should not be the main focus of care until it has been demonstrated that they work. He concludes that while it is theoretically possible to do away with mental hospitals altogether by treating every mental patient in the community, there is no assurance that community treatment will prevent chronic disability altogether.

Nevertheless, Wing is not pessimistic about the community mental health approach. He believes that the general emphasis in this direction has had an overall beneficial effect upon the approaches to treatment of mental patients. Ongoing studies of the community mental health approaches continue to be conducted by Wing and his Medical Research Council Social Psychiatry Unit at the Maudsley, focused upon the activities of the Maudsley services to its own Camberwell catchment area. Wing feels that such service responsibility is important if an institution is to carry out properly its teaching and research responsibilities.

At the time of my visit, Wing was involved in a study of patients from the Camberwell catchment area who had been out of touch with a psychiatrist for over a year and was also studying the effectiveness of rehabilitation for psychotic patients who had not worked for at least a year. Half of the index cases under study are controls; the other half (the study population) are admitted to the rehabilitation programs of the day hospital at the Maudsley. There is great emphasis on "rehabilitation through work" in the community mental health programs in Britain, and both the St. Francis and Maudsley day hospital programs include a rehabilitation workshop or industrial therapy unit. Wing feels that for such rehabilitative programs to be effective, it is necessary to maintain a close relationship with the specialist vocational expert at the local employment exchange, who is instrumental in finding employment for handicapped workers. He also advocates close ties with the housing and welfare authorities.

I attended a research session of the rehabilitation study at which both Dr. John Wing and Dr. Lorna Wing were present, in addition to a clinical psychologist, Mr. Griffiths, and a social scientist, Dr. Stevens. The function of the latter is to interview the relatives and make measurements of the social background. The patient is examined by Dr. Lorna Wing and is tested by the psychologist. Criteria for inclusion in the study are that the patient is a male between the ages of 20 and 55 who has been diagnosed as psychotic, and who has been unable to remain regularly employed. Half of the patients are then assigned to the control group and the other half to the experimental group. However, participation in the rehabilitation program by the experimental group is voluntary, so that not all patients so assigned actually participate. Approximately 75 patients in all had been worked up, of whom 35 actually entered the control or experimental groups. Evaluative studies of this kind, together with the Camberwell Register, account for about half of the unit's research activities.

The Outpatient Program

The Maudsley conducts an active outpatient program, and there is a large psychotherapy department. It is not common for outpatient programs of British hospitals to offer large-scale intensive psychotherapy, and the Maudsley has had the reputation of being organic rather than psychodynamic in its orientation; indeed, the institution has been accused in the United States of antipsychoanalytic views. Therefore, the fact that psychotherapy has for many years been offered regularly at the Maudsley deserves some note.

The term "psychotherapy" refers to group therapy as well as intensive individual psychotherapy. It reaches only a small proportion of the total community, particularly in the Camberwell area, because the necessity for prolonged treatment means that it is restricted to relatively few patients. On the other hand, combinations of supportive psychotherapy and drugs are used for about 13% of the outpatient caseload who are seen for regular appointments weekly or monthly for an average of 20 visits per year. The remainder of the outpatients are seen for approximately five or six visits and then discharged. Some patients are treated on a regular, continuing basis with drugs without supportive psychotherapy.

In the Adult Outpatient Department there is a clinic for problems of forensic psychiatry; most of the patients are referred from magistrates' courts or from probation officers. The daytime clinic is supplemented by two evening clinics. In the Children's Outpatient Department a clinic is run for problems of juvenile delinquency. Patients requiring treatment are taken on by the registrars under the consultant's supervision. The hospital also supplies a diagnostic service to the London Remand Home for boys, the Remand Prison at Brixton, and the Hospital Prison at Gremdon.

The Maudsley also operates a 24-hour, 7-day-a-week emergency service which is extensively used; but technically speaking, the proper procedure under the health service is for psychiatric emergencies to go first to their general practitioner, who would then be expected to refer them to the proper facility for treatment. In practice, however, a number of patients present themselves directly at the hospital outpatient service without prior referral from the general practitioner.

Cooperation between the hospital and the local authority varies widely in different vicinities. The Maudsley's relationship with the local authorities responsible for their catchment area has been fairly close, particularly in the spheres of social welfare, housing, and education. This close relationship evolved out of the careful planning and preparation that took place before the Maudsley took over responsibility for the Camberwell catchment area. However, the relationship has been altered by the Social Services Act (Seebohm), which takes mental health social work from the control of the Medical Officer of Health and combines it in a new Social Service Department (101). There are no longer any distinctions between health, mental welfare, child welfare, or other welfare services. These services are now being distributed in the area in district offices.

The Maudsley Day Hospital

The Day Hospital at the Maudsley is located on the opposite side of the grounds from the Institute of Psychiatry. Dr. Douglas Bennett is in charge of this program, which has 36 places in the Day Hospital proper, and a like number at the adjoining Industrial Rehabilitation Unit (IRU). In addition, Dr. Bennett is responsible for approximately 60 patients at St. Francis Hospital and also for a few beds at Cane Hill.

The Day Hospital is operated with a distinctly medical orientation. There are three young doctors (two registrars, one clinical assistant); three psychiatric nurses; two social workers; one occupational therapist; and a part-time clinical psychologist. There are also several clinical psychology students, social work students, and occupational therapy students. The staff is organized around three clinical teams, with one doctor nominally at the head of each. However, this leadership is more in name than in fact, since the doctors rotate every three months, while the other staff remain more or less permanently.

Each clinical team meets several times weekly to discuss the patients assigned to them, approximately 12 per team. There is another meeting at which all clinical teams meet for "supervision" by a psychoanalyst, whose function it is to further communication among staff members and to help them to make direct interpretations of the patients' behavior to the patients. In addition, each clinical team meets jointly with the patients for whom it is responsible, and there is also one general meeting each week where both teams and patients meet with Bennett.

The social workers work a great deal with the patients' families, particularly when the patients are becoming ready to find employment, but only infrequently with the patients themselves. The occupational therapist supervises the work program in which the patients participate when they are not attending meetings. The doctors administer electroshock therapy, prescribe drugs, and "supervise" the clinical teams in their approach to their assigned patients.

The Industrial Rehabilitation Unit (IRU) also has an occupational therapist, but in addition, there is an industrial rehabilitation expert from industry. Both the Day Hospital proper and the IRU do contract work, but the work done at the Day Hospital Unit has a much lower level of aspiration and is done under much less pressure. In the IRU, the staff seek to simulate the conditions of industry; patients have to be on time, they have to turn out work of high quality, etc. The Day Hospital is looked upon as a stepping stone to the IRU. In contrast to the Day Hospital, there is no medical emphasis at the IRU, the entire emphasis being social and occupational. In fact, the doctors usually do not even visit the IRU, nor are there nurses about. The social workers, however, continue to be active with the families of patients in the IRU.

Most of the patients at the Day Hospital have been referred by Maudsley, Bethlem Royal, or St. Francis hospitals, following a period of inpatient stay. However, a certain number are admitted directly following evaluation in the outpatient clinic. These are usually chronic patients, many of whom have had numerous hospital admissions. Because of Dr. Wing's rehabilitation study of patients without regular employment, this type of severely handicapped patient made up the major portion of the patient population at the Day Hospital at the time of my visit. Several of the patients had not worked more than three months over the previous ten years. About one third of the population were diagnosed as chronic schizophrenics, with the remainder labeled as having severe character disorders, particularly of the inadequate type.

The Day Hospital and the IRU occupy buildings side by side, each in an old, reconverted house, with three floors above ground and a basement level below. All floors are utilized. In the Day Hospital, there are offices for the doctors on the top floor, and also the office of Dr. Bennett's secretary. On the floor below are Bennett's office and several patients' activity rooms.

At the time I visited, patients were doing clerical work in one of the rooms; in another, they were producing parts of a tailor's dummy. The latter work consisted of winding and twisting wires and joining them at an appropriate place. The floor below contains additional workshop areas, as well as a patients' lounge where the group meetings are held. There is also a reception area on this floor and the office of the sister in charge of the Day Hospital. The ground floor, or basement level, contains additional workshop areas, where patients were engaged in a variety of light-type industrial activities, such as folding toy balloons and stuffing them into plastic envelopes. Some of the patients were obviously deficient intellectually, in addition to their other handicaps.

The Industrial Rehabilitation Unit

The Industrial Rehabilitation Unit next door has about the same physical structure as the Day Hospital but is equipped for heavier types of industrial work. There is a machine shop where metal turning is done. One project in the woodworking area at the time of my visit was the production of the popular device with five suspended steel balls, used to illustrate the conservation of momentum, which can be derived from Newton's Second Law. In another room patients were preparing graphs to illustrate some of the research being done at the Institute of Psychiatry. In another area a patient was typing mimeograph stencils for a scientific article, including bibliography, written by one of the staff; in yet another area, one patient was checking the IBM card-punching which was being done by another patient on an IBM card-punching machine. Two other such machines in the same room were not being utilized at the time.

In another room, patients were engaged in making electrical devices such as heating equipment, a thermostat for fish aquaria, and an infrared heating unit. I noticed another area, equipped with various kinds of duplicating machines, which serves as a print shop. There is an office for the industrial manager and another for the occupational therapist. The atmosphere in both buildings is friendly and cheerful. The patients seem to be in a good humor even when they acknowledge that they have not worked in the past ten years.

Bennett stated that between them, the units have had 30-40% success in finding jobs for these chronic, unemployed people. Others, who had spent years in the hospital, have been placed in the community with their families even though they are able to work only in sheltered workshops operated by the Department of Employment and Productivity, or to remain idle at home. The patient in the community also has the option of attending some day centers operated by the local authority.

Bennett sees the Day Hospital as but one part of the total therapeutic spectrum. He considers it difficult to evaluate its effectiveness since it is not doing the entire job, and definitive results can only be obtained through the wide-scale interaction of the various treatment units of the total. Bennett feels that the emphasis upon working with families has not taken hold as much in England as it has in the United States, possibly because of the difference in attitude of the English people towards such involvement. They tend to see the psychiatric patient as someone apart and distinct from themselves and tend to separate themselves sharply from him as if to indicate that he is sick, they are well, and consequently, they don't need to see anybody.

While many day hospitals send psychiatric nurses into the community to visit patients in their homes, Bennett prefers that the patients visit the hospital and see the nurses there, feeling that this is much more efficient in terms of time.

Bennett worked with Maxwell Jones in the original therapeutic-community project and sees what he is now doing as a modification of that program. He has traveled widely and has visited industrial therapy projects as far afield as Copenhagen and Buenos Aires. He lectured on British psychiatry at the 1973 Annual Meeting of the American Psychiatric Association (APA) in Honolulu.

Teaching and Research

The Institute of Psychiatry functions as an autonomous unit of the University of London. It is concerned primarily with postgraduate education and is not connected with any undergraduate medical school except informally. The institute maintains departments in the basic sciences of biochemistry, physiology, psychology, and biometrics under the same roof as the clinical Department of Psychiatry. In addition, there is a longstanding Department of Neuropathology, as well as a new Department of Neurology established jointly by the institute and Kings College Hospital Medical School in 1972. During the 1969-70 academic year, 469 postgraduate students obtained training at the Institute of Psychiatry (as compared with 417 in the previous year). This figure does not include part-time students who spend two months or less there. Several kinds of degrees are offered, including Ph.D., M.Sc., M. Phil., and M. Phil. in Psychiatry. The latter has now replaced the D.P.M. as the designation of completion of postgraduate psychiatric studies. The last of the D.P.M. examinations was given at the University of London in April 1969.

There are increasing numbers of students in psychiatry who come from other countries. Two hundred-ten, of whom 66 were new arrivals, were enrolled for the academic year 1970-71, coming from over 50 different countries. The largest single national contingent was from the United States (26), followed by India (22), Canada (19), Pakistan (16), and Australia (13). The foreign doctors are usually sponsored by their home countries and supported by grants or scholarships from their own governments or from groups such as the World Health Organization, the British Council, the Association of Commonwealth Universities, or from other grant-giving bodies.

Because of the increasing number of students, special efforts are being made to provide for their special needs. For example, to facilitate acquisition of suitable living accommodations for these visiting doctors, a limited number of single rooms have been leased at a comparatively low rent in a new staff hostel on the Maudsley campus. The hostel, Princess Marina House, otherwise provides accommodation primarily for nursing staff. Also, a special series of seminars and tutorials for overseas students was recently instituted.

The international atmosphere is reflected in the roster of visiting lecturers, as well as by the student body. Again, the United States is the most well represented. For example, the first Aubrey Lewis Lecture was given by Dr. Lawrence C. Kolb, of Columbia University, in November 1969.

In the area of research in psychiatry, a major undertaking is a joint United States-United Kingdom diagnostic project comparing patterns of psychiatric diagnosis in the two countries (99). This is a long-term study supported by the National Institute of Mental Health. Other projects include a study of the treatment of autistic children, supported by the Department of Health and Social Security; the classification of mental disorders, supported by the World Health Organization; as well as a number of Medical Research Council supported projects, including studies of factors affecting memory in depressed patients, the treatment of phobias, normal versus disturbed adolescent boys, epidemiological studies of epilepsy in subnormal children, and studies of various aspects of brain activity in monkeys. These investigations are in addition to those already described, such as Wing's studies and Camberwell Register. Two Medical Research Council units are housed at the institute: the Social Psychiatry Research Unit, and the Psychiatric Genetics Research Unit.

Active research programs are also conducted by the institute's departments of biochemistry, biometrics, neuropathology, physiology, and psychology. In the latter department, the name best known in the United States is probably that of Professor H. J. Eysenck, a behaviorist who has written extensively on evaluation of psychotherapy (24, 25). His current investigations include studies of social and sexual attitudes in relation to personality variables.

13

Community mental health services for a London borough: Camden

The London Council Reorganization of 1964-65 created Camden Borough as a heterogeneous amalgam of districts with a gerrymandered shape, encompassing a population of 240,000. Camden contains three railroad stations (Euston, St. Pancras, Kings Cross), several major teaching hospitals (University College Hospital, Royal Free Hospital), two major psychoanalytic/psychiatric centers (Tavistock Centre, Hampstead Clinic), a small part of the east boundary of Regents Park (up to, but not including the zoo), the University of London, and the British Museum. There are 75 schools and institutions of higher learning, research establishments, and specialized schools, both public and private, within the borough. There are 34 hospitals, including nursing homes, a veterinary hospital, and a specialized hospital for otolaryngology. There is also a day unit for autistic children, formerly operated by the section on Maternal and Child Care of the Health Department, but now the responsibility of the new Social Service Department.

The borough includes the neighborhoods of South, East, and West Hampstead; Swiss Cottage; Kentish Town; Chalk Farm; Camden Town; and Bloomsbury. It is a borough in transition and includes a large transient population. Several neighborhoods have undergone marked physical alteration, such as Bloomsbury and Swiss Cottage, both of which have been significantly upgraded as a result of urban renewal and other efforts. But there are still more rooming houses (bedsitters) than apartments (flats)

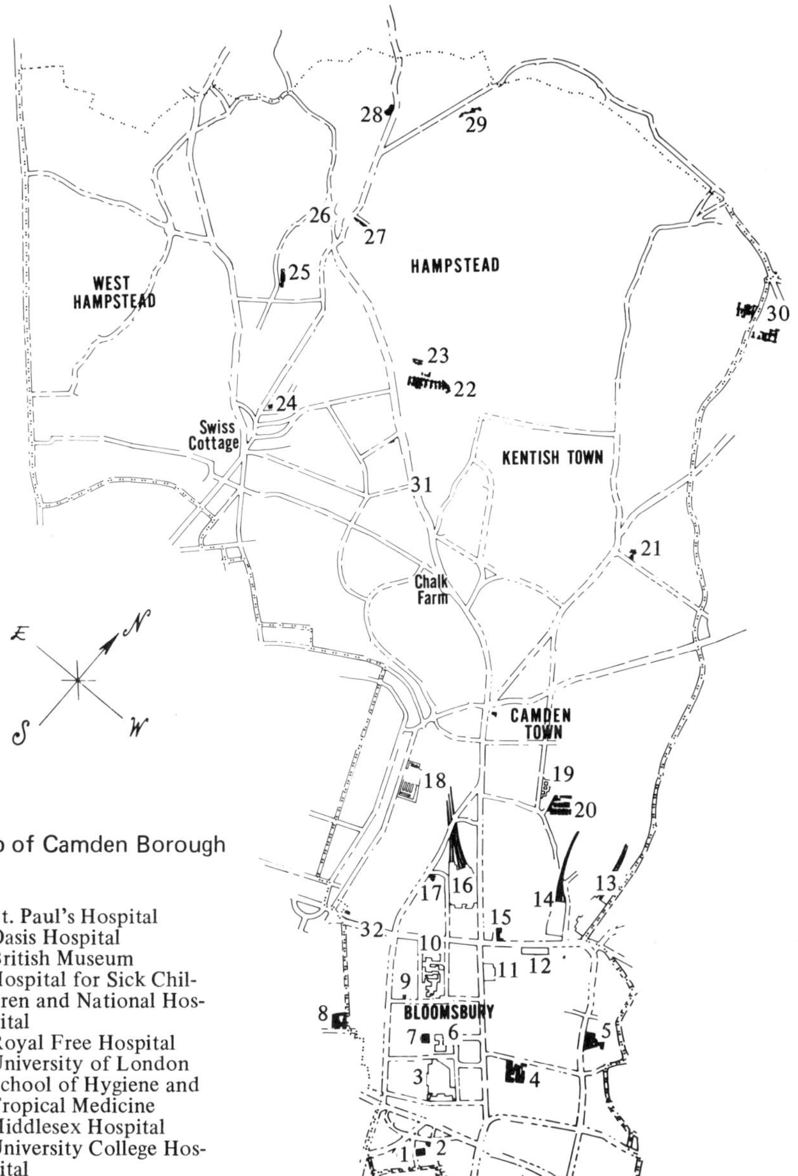

Map of Camden Borough

1. St. Paul's Hospital
2. Oasis Hospital
3. British Museum
4. Hospital for Sick Children and National Hospital
5. Royal Free Hospital
6. University of London
7. School of Hygiene and Tropical Medicine
8. Middlesex Hospital
9. University College Hospital
10. University College
11. British Medical Association
12. Bidborough House
13. Kings Cross Station
14. St. Pancras Station
15. Elizabeth Garrett Anderson Hospital
16. Euston Station
17. National Temple Hospital
18. Regents Park Barracks and Hospital
19. Royal Veterinary College
20. St. Pancras Hospital
21. St. Margaret's Hospital
22. Royal Free Hospital
23. Hampstead General Hospital
24. Tavistock Institute
25. University College School
26. Medical Research Institute
27. New End Hospital
28. Manor Home Hospital (Women)
29. St. Colombus Hospital
30. Whittington Hospital
31. Haverstock Hill Road
32. Euston Road

and more flats than houses. A large student population lives around the university. There are numerous hotels around Russell Square and Tavistock Square, and many transients live near the railroad stations. The population is heterogeneous and includes numerous immigrant groups: German-Jewish refugees; an older group and a more recent group of immigrants from Ireland; Indian, Pakistani, and West Indian communities; some Africans; and a number of Cypriots. The borough was such an unlikely conglomerate that many expected at its creation that it would not work. This challenge, however, made the Borough Council more determined than ever to make it work and paradoxically gave rise to attitudes that have made Camden Borough among the most progressive in London.

The immigrant groups have tended to cluster in enclaves within the borough and, for the most part, have remained segregated from the surrounding communities. Thus, the German-Jewish refugees (chiefly World War II refugees who now constitute an older age group) have collected around Hampstead; the Cypriots have settled in Kentish Town, etc. The Irish immigrants, the older group as well as the new arrivals, are distinctly outsiders. The West Indian immigrants are probably the most "English" because of their cultural familiarity with the traditional institutions, but they suffer the usual prejudices because of their black skin. The Pakistani are probably in the lowest sociocultural echelon. They are chiefly unskilled laborers who work very hard and are viewed as an economic threat on this count by the native unskilled workers. The Indians are likewise industrious but tend to be involved in business and shopkeeping. The handful of Africans living in Camden have come to Britain chiefly to study. This group includes couples, both of whom are enrolled in schools of various kinds, who present a problem because they have children whom they place in foster homes. This practice is in keeping with a characteristic African pattern of having children raised by the extended family rather than by the parents; but because of the social differences here, the extended family role is replaced by foster homes which are often not of high quality. Foster homes represent an expense to the community and create difficulties and friction because of dissatisfaction with the care given to the children.

The Cypriots are the most internally cohesive group. The women usually do not even speak English, although the men, because they work among English-speaking people, generally know some English. Unlike other clannish groups, however, they do not look after their own social and economic problems, nor does the Greek Orthodox Church provide for the social needs of these people. Consequently, the community and the Council of Social Services have in recent years been called upon to provide service for this group. Their efforts have been fraught with difficulty, because the Cypriots' culture makes assimilation into the surrounding milieu difficult.

Generally, the socio-economic status of Camden Borough is low. The concentration of railroad stations in the borough probably accounts for the large number of transients, many of them down-and-outers and derelicts, who live near the stations. A few areas have reached rock bottom, have been rehabilitated, and are now on the upgrade socioeconomically. For example, Hampstead is being converted from bedsitters to rather expensive flats.

The emphasis of the community mental health programs in Camden, as elsewhere throughout Britain, is largely upon posthospital aftercare, rehabilitation, and resocialization services. Voluntary organizations generally provide such preventive efforts as there are. There is a high tolerance in the community for eccentricity, as there is throughout England, and patients may reach advanced stages of illness before they are brought to the attention of their general practitioner, or before the general practitioner sees fit to refer the patient to a psychiatric consultant for admission to the mental hospital.

Once the patient is identified as mentally ill, he is usually admitted to Friern Hospital, but at times patients may be admitted to one of the two teaching hospitals in the borough (University College Hospital or Royal Free Hospital), or to Middlesex Hospital, a teaching hospital just north of Camden. Most patients are discharged and returned to the community after a relatively short time. Those coming from the teaching hospitals are provided with aftercare and casework counseling by the local-authority social work staff. Those discharged from the mental hospital receive aftercare services at outpatient clinics operated by the mental hospital, or they may be referred to either of two day centers operated by the local authority. They may also become members of one of the therapeutic social clubs in the borough operated either by local authority or voluntary auspices. There are no sheltered worshops or hostels in the borough, and patients in need of such accommodations must be referred elsewhere. An effort has been made to link together and integrate the services provided by the mental hospital, the teaching hospitals, and the local authority, but this linkage is fairly loose and communication between the various elements is not very good.

LOCAL AUTHORITY SERVICES

The Medical Officer of Health for Camden Borough is Dr. Wilfred Harding, who came to Camden at its inception in 1965. Consequently, he is the only MOH the borough has had. Dr. Harding has apparently been interested in the problems of mental health for some time but had been prevented from implementing his ideas in his previous post by the frugality of the Borough Council. When he found that the council was ready and willing to support him, he was determined to make an effective program. Harding points out that the Camden Borough Council is quite unusual, as councils go. For example, members have contributed money from their own pockets to make up deficits that resulted from their undercharging of rents to tenants in the housing developments.

Harding set up a program which involved the mental hospitals, the teaching hospital (University College Hospital), and the Local Authority Public Health Service. Dr. Bernard Adams, the consultant psychiatrist, holds a joint appointment with the Local Authority Health Department, Friern Hospital, and University College Hospital. Harding told me that this is the only tripartite arrangement of this sort in London.

At the time of my first visit, the borough was faced with a number of difficulties, one of which was a built-in division of responsibility which made the comprehensiveness of services sought by Harding impossible to achieve. For example, the provision of mental health services was compartmentalized and fragmented within the local authority structure. Services for children were provided by the Children's Department, unless there were educational aspects, in which case they were provided by the Education Department. The latter includes child guidance programs, which are considered educational rather than psychiatric, although the Education Department does employ psychiatrists, as well as psychologists and social workers, in its guidance clinics. Services for the mentally subnormal, traditionally the responsibility of the Health Department, were also scheduled to be moved to the Education Department. Problems pertaining to displacement of families, as a consequence of "urban renewal" programs that resulted in changes of living accommodations, were the province of the Housing Department, although such upheavals are frequently accompanied by emotional stress. Similarly, emotional difficulties surrounding the economic hardships of families were expected to be dealt with in the Welfare Department.

Another division of responsibility stemmed from the fact that the catchment area population of 240,000 was served by two mental hospitals (Horton Hospital and Friern Hospital) so that there was no clear-cut correspondence of the local authority's area of responsibility with those of the mental hospitals. Most of the catchment area was served by Friern Hospital; the Hampstead area was served by Horton Hospital. Recently, this difficulty was corrected, when Friern Hospital assumed responsibility for the entire borough. Even today, however, some Camden patients are hospitalized at one or another of the teaching hospitals.

Patients who are discharged from the mental hospital are not followed by the local-authority social work staff. Instead, they are seen at the outpatient clinics operated by the mental hospital. On the other hand, the social workers from the local authority will follow patients discharged from the University College Hospital, Royal Free Hospital, and Middlesex Hospital. The local-authority social workers do not have a good working relationship with the social workers from the mental hospital, though they would like to. Possibly the hospital social workers may feel threatened by the local authority staff, or vice versa. According to Harding, they do try to work closely with the Council of Social Services and with volunteer groups in the borough, but there is no organized procedure for doing so.

Another problem stems from the social workers' definition of their role. For example, the social workers of the local authority work only with patients who have been diagnosed as mentally ill. If they suspect that a person is mentally ill, they may refer him to the general practitioner and suggest that a psychiatric evaluation be made. At other times, they may not, since their main emphasis is not on primary prevention or early case-finding, but rather on posthospital care or rehabilitation. They tend to "nurse" the patient in the community by helping him with his personal problems and by increasing the general tolerance of the patient by the community. They do not look upon their service as therapeutic, considering that the responsibiligy for providing therapeutic service lies with the hospital.

The effectiveness of the tripartite arrangement between the local authority, mental hospital, and teaching hospital was further impaired when the recommendations of the Seebohm Report went into effect. Prior to 1971, the principal social worker in the mental health section of the local authority was Miss P. M. Perrott, and 18 social workers worked under her. Of these, 7 were fully qualified psychiatric social workers, while the others were medical social workers and partially trained people. All social workers in the mental health section functioned as MWOs, in addition to carrying their usual case work responsibilities.

Since the implementation of the Seebohm Report, with social workers from the Children's Department, Welfare Department, and mental health section of the Health Department combined into a single Department of Social Services, Harding's responsibilities for child care, welfare, and mental health have been absorbed by the new department. The new director is Kenneth Urwin, and there are now 90 social workers in the Social Service Department. The largest single contingent came from the Children's Department, the second largest group was from the Welfare Department, and the smallest group consisted of the 18 mental health workers who were looked upon as an "elite corps" because of the generally higher level of their training. Without regard for their background or experience, the social workers have been assigned administratively to one of five subcatchment areas; each area group contains 18 workers. Only the group in Kentish Town actually work in the community. They are the most satisfied group, because they are less involved with administrative problems and interact more with clientele in the field. Their offices are based at the Lodge on Leighton Road. The offices of the remaining four area groups (Holborn and Somers Town, Regents Park, West Hampstead, and Grafton) are located at Bidborough House, a good-sized, fairly modern building located just off Euston Road, not far from the railroad stations.

The Social Service Department is now responsible for both the mentally subnormal and the mentally ill. While it has mandatory responsibility for all of the mentally subnormal, it can be somewhat selective in providing services for the mentally ill. On Thursday mornings Dr. Adams consults with the four groups at Bidborough House; the Kentish group usually does not attend. Adams finds communication with these groups difficult, because most of the workers are not interested in mental health problems. A number of the more experienced workers from the mental health section have left the borough to accept better-paying administrative positions elsewhere. The remaining workers are less well trained and have no background in mental health. The overall quality of the social workers has therefore declined.

Miss Perrott, formerly the principal social worker in the mental health section, now in charge of the West Hampstead area, is responsible for children, welfare, and the aged. She reflects the general dissatisfaction with the overall approach of the new department. In essence, she finds that the conflict is sharpest between the traditional welfare approach and that of the trained psychiatric social worker. An underlying problem is the rivalry between the better-trained PSW and the many less well trained workers coming from the other departments.

Although there are plans to redistribute the MWO's responsibilities, the psychiatric social workers are still carrying out these commitments. The requirement that the MWO be on emergency call for a 24-hour period makes the task particularly unattractive to the social workers who lack a psychiatric background, despite the extra pay involved. One worker from each of the five areas rotates this duty on a daily basis, covering the entire borough. Therefore the borough is not compartmentalized into areas as far as the MWO's function is concerned. There has been, however, some redistribution of other responsibilities. For example, all of the day centers in the borough, including those for children, old people, mentally retarded adults, and mentally ill (the Lyndhurst and Raydon Centres) have been placed under the jurisdiction of one person, Mrs. Jessica Brill, formerly a child-care worker. The Raydon Centre, providing industrial therapy, and the Lyndhurst Centre, providing occupational therapy, are housed in space donated to the Health Department; both are staffed by paid nonprofessionals. Most of the staff have no special skills or background, although two of the four staff members of the Raydon Centre do have industrial experience. The staff-to-patient ratio in each center is approximately one to ten.

Raydon Centre

Raydon Centre was opened in 1967 in an old building which was previously a glue factory. There are plans to establish a purpose-built center. There were four staff members, two men and two women, at the time of my first visit. Mr. Rowlands, in charge of the industrial work program, has a background in industry. He is assisted by Mr. James, who has had experience in industrial psychology and some hospital experience with the physically disabled. Miss Margaret Carr was previously a psychiatric nurse, and the other female staff member is an occupational therapist who also has a background in psychiatric nursing. They were trying to obtain a fifth staff member.

The center originally expected to provide places for 35 patients, but in practice, the maximum that they can normally handle is 25. The patients attend five days per week, between 9:00 A.M. and 4:00 P.M. Attendance is normally good, but if someone fails to attend, a follow-up is made either by a call directly from the center, or through one of the social workers of the local authority. The social workers maintain contact with all of the patients in the center, including those from the mental hospital. The proportion of male to female patients varies. The age of the patients ranges between 17 and 55 years but most are between the ages of 30 and 40. Some of the patients who find outside employment may fail and subsequently return to the center, but these are in the minority. The center operates a social club on Wednesday evenings, which was being moved to the premises of the Camden Association of Mental Health at the time of my visit. There were plans to start another club on Thursday evening.

The center has facilities for carrying out light industrial projects. Contracts are made with outside firms, who supply the machines and equipment needed to carry out their projects. The activities vary. On the upper floor of the center, twelve patients are normally engaged in light industrial activities, such as packing table-tennis fittings or toys, making paint boxes, etc. On the lower floor is a machine shop, which also is capable of handling light engineering work. Projects here include making electrician's tape or table-tennis fittings, which are packed upstairs. The rate of production in the machine shop is about half the rate expected of outside industrial firms. Patients work six hours a day in the center, as opposed to the normal 8-hour industrial day. The standard of work is high, and there are few rejects. The patients are required to clock in, and are strictly supervised as to the time taken for tea breaks and lunch, in order to simulate industrial working conditions as much as possible.

When work is contracted for with an industrial firm, a price is negotiated for each job. The base pay for a patient is 25 new pence per day, plus car fare and social security. This amount may be increased to 39 new pence, depending upon the patient's productivity.

Most patients are referred by psychiatrists from the catchment area's mental hospitals, while others are referred by general practitioners or by social workers of the local authority. Placing patients in the Raydon Centre, as well as the Lyndhurst Centre, is now a complicated process. Mrs. Brill is not accustomed to working with problems of mental patients, and there is a great deal of dissatisfaction and confusion on all sides.

At the time of my first visit, four patients at the center were still residents at the mental hospital and were preparing for discharge. They traveled to and fro between the center and the hospital each day. The average length of stay at the center was between two and three months. The shortest recorded stay was six weeks, the longest, 18 months. Some patients do poorly and must be returned to the hospital. Most patients at the center live in the community with their families, a few live in psychiatric hostels, and a few live on their own. Although there are no psychiatric hostels in Camden Borough, there is one in the neighboring borough of Barnett, in which some Camden patients have been placed.

Food for the midday meal is provided by meals-on-wheels from the town hall. The patients eat in a canteen operated by the center and supervised by a staff member with the assistance of two patients. The center owns its own cutlery, dishes, etc. Dishwashing is done by the two patients. The center was planning to start a program for cooking, shopping, and care of personal garments, but this had not yet been initiated at the time of my visit.

Two group meetings are held for the patients each week, one for the more articulate patients, the other for the less articulate. These are attended by social workers from the local authority.

Although the Raydon Centre is located on the very edge of Camden Borough, and public transportation to the center is poor, attendance is very good. Most patients are on medication, and the medicines are normally held by the center staff and issued to the patients at scheduled times. Medication is prescribed at the outpatient clinics operated by the mental hospital.

Lyndhurst Day Centre

The Lyndhurst Day Centre is housed in a very old building located in the middle of a Council Estate of new flats.* In addition to its

*Council Estates are public housing projects. These may consist of individual dwellings (Council Houses) or apartment buildings (blocks of flats.)

use as a day center, the building is rented out for such activities as a youth club, an old peoples club, and a boxing club. The day center also operates a Thursday Evening (therapeutic) Social Club on the premises. Financial support for both the Raydon and Lyndhurst centers is provided by the Camden Borough Local Authority, supplemented by grants from the Ministry of Health. The Borough Council even paid the cost of a one-week seaside holiday for the staff and patients of the center.

There are only two staff members at the Lyndhurst Centre. John Bennett, the supervisor, is a former commercial-art student with previous experience working at an industrial day center at Islington. He was assisted by Elizabeth Swinson, an American who had been in Britain only nine months at the time of my visit. She was formerly a psychology student and had worked with disturbed children. Miss Swinson had been at the center for six months and Mr. Bennett for five months at the time of my visit. Before Bennett arrived, the center staff had always been exclusively female.

The center provides places for 20 patients, but the number who actually attend varies. When I visited the center, 18 patients were enrolled, with an average daily attendance of 14. The Lyndhurst Centre, run on much less strict lines than the Raydon Centre, tries both to create a sense of responsibility in the patients and to broaden their outlook, particularly with respect to social and interpersonal relationships.

Activities include sports, music, painting, cooking, talking, reading books, and playing a variety of games including draughts (checkers), chess, and cards. The paid staff of the center are assisted by three volunteers, each of whom provides specialized services for the patients. One of the volunteers teaches English; another conducts dramatic interpretations, drama classes, and speech classes; while the third conducts classes in dance and movements. In the summer patients play tennis in the local park, and an outing is usually arranged once a week to places of interest, such as zoos or parks. The staff were also planning a "quiet room" where patients may escape from the group if they wish. A formal group meeting is held weekly; there is usually a second, more informal one.

The patients decide among themselves what their luncheon menu will be, do their own marketing, and prepare the food in the center's kitchen. The daily budget is 15 new pence per person, and the meals must be planned around this budgetary limitation. Specific assignments such as marketing, cooking, and serving food are shared among the patients.

The age range of patients is between 17 and 45 years, but most are between the ages of 20 and 30. Most of the patients take medication, but unlike the Raydon Centre, Lyndhurst allows patients to keep their own medicines. For the most part, attendance is good and, as at Raydon

Centre, follow-ups are made on patients who fail to attend regularly. The majority of patients are single and live in rooms in government hostels, which, as previously noted, are outside of the borough, since Camden operates no hostels of its own. Few patients live with their families. The length of stay at Lyndhurst varies between two and six months.

Most of the patients at Lyndhurst are unemployed and are receiving social security benefits. Their carfare to and from the center is paid by the Borough Council. The social workers of the mental health section maintain contact with all of the patients.

Patients at the center are accepted on a selective basis, mainly from among those discharged from the mental hospital. Patients also may be referred to the center by the general practitioner, social worker, or a relative; it is not essential that the patient be seen by a psychiatrist. If it is felt that a patient cannot be helped at the center, he may be sent to an alternative agency that might be able to assist him. For example, aged people are not considered suitable for admission to the Lyndhurst Centre. A major criterion for selection is the patient's own desire for community care after his discharge from the mental hospital. Occasionally, a patient may go to the center before he is actually discharged from the hospital. The local-authority social workers maintain contact with the psychiatrist in the hospital, who serves as consultant to the social workers when they have questions about the patients' behavior or their management. However, the psychiatric consultant may be called out to visit the patients, by the general practitioner only, not by the social workers.

A few patients retain friendships formed at the center, but sometimes the patients do not get along with one another. Physical fights between patients at the center have occurred, as well as suicide or attempted suicide. Occasionally, the patients become sexually involved with one another. However, the center staff tend not to discourage sexual involvement, and sometimes even encourage it as a means of establishing some basis for interpersonal communication between the patients.

During my first visit I attended a Bidborough House conference at which there was a case presentation of a patient being seen at the Lyndhurst Centre, who had formerly been at the Raydon Centre. Those attending included the central social work staff of the mental health section of the Health Department, some of the staff from the day centers, and Dr. Bernard Adams, the consultant psychiatrist. I was the only outsider, except for a student from the Tavistock.

The patient was, of course, not present. He was a man of Rumanian birth, who refused to take medication and was subject to periodic paranoid outbursts. He obviously required a great deal of external structure and, in fact, his paranoid symptoms regularly became most manifest just prior to weekends, when he would be on his own. He had left the Raydon Centre for two reasons: he could not relate socially to the other patients and he resented having to conform to the industrial therapy program. Paradoxically, he seemed to do much better at the Lyndhurst Centre where there is much less structure, and the pressures to conform are much less strict. The report indicated that the patient had established a good relationship with Mr. Bennett, the supervisor of the Lyndhurst Centre. The discussion of the case by the staff reflected a lively interest in and considerable understanding of the problems presented by the patient.

The effectiveness of the Lyndhurst Centre has been challenged by the new Social Service Department staff, who feel that Lyndhurst is not performing efficiently enough to justify costs.

HOSPITAL SERVICES

Responsibility for the majority of Camden Borough's population of 240,000 rests with the Friern Hospital, located in Barnett, in the northwestern part of London. A typical Victorian institution, surrounded by spacious grounds, it was built in 1860 as a 2,800-bed mental hospital, of which 2,200 beds are now occupied. At the time of its construction it was rather distant from the center of London's population, but the institution has now become completely engulfed by the spread of urban development.

Initially the Friern Hospital catchment area covered a wide sector of London, including Islington and most of Camden Borough, except for Hampstead. Hampstead was served by the Horton Mental Hospital, located in Epsom. This gave rise to some confusion and administrative difficulties. Friern Hospital has recently assumed responsibility for the entire borough, which greatly facilitates administrative procedures.

Friern Hospital was initially organized in almost every respect along traditional lines. The buildings were sexually segregated, with those housing women patients arranged along one side of the administration building and those housing the men patients along the opposite side. Many of the hospital wards were locked, and there were typical back wards housing the most deteriorated patients. These patients did not have access to the hospital grounds, and there was no provision for occupational or industrial therapy. According to Adams, two new experimental wards were completed in 1971 in a remodeled portion of the male wing to house 40 to 50 patients. This represents the hospital's first experiment with a ward for patients of both sexes. The experimental unit is well staffed and is used for intensive therapy for acute patients. There are now buildings on the grounds for industrial therapy, occupational therapy, and related programs shared by patients from various wards in the hospital. In addition, there is a ward at nearby Halliwick Hospital, which also has a very high staff-to-patient ratio and a very intensive treatment program. Halliwick concentrates on the less seriously ill, more neurotic patient.

The six psychiatric consultants at Friern are organized into three clinical teams or "firms," with three or four registrars assigned to each team. The responsibility is fairly evenly divided; each consultant is in charge of some acute wards on one wing and some chronic wards on the other.

There are approximately 2,000 admissions and discharges per year. The average length of stay for the majority of new admissions is around 30 days, although the most chronically ill patients may remain in the hospital for years. The majority of the hospital beds continue to be occupied by such long-stay patients.

The number of nurses at the hospital is quite limited. Many of the chronic wards are short-staffed, and the quality of the staff is uneven. The acute units tend to be somewhat better staffed. While all types of therapy are available, the greatest reliance seems to be placed on drugs. It was my impression that Dr. Adams employs electroshock treatment less frequently than do many of his colleagues.

Some of the patients from Camden Borough may alternatively be hospitalized in the teaching hospitals such as the Royal Free Hospital, University College Hospital, or Middlesex Hospital. While the University College Hospital has an inpatient unit of 60 psychiatric beds in the main hospital, most of the psychiatric patients from Camden are sent to the St. Pancras Hospital, which is affiliated with the University College Hospital and which contains a poor-law unit of 56 beds divided between male and female wings in the traditional pattern. Adams, the Friern consultant, admits acute patients who seem to have the best chances for rapid return to the community, to the St. Pancras unit, provided a bed is available. The remainder are admitted to Friern. For a time St. Pancras Hospital assumed responsibility for a segment of the Camden catchment area, but the attempt failed, because its resources were insufficient and it lacked supportive facilities, such as day hospitals, outpatient treatment activities, hostels, sheltered workshops, etc. The projected ratio was one-half bed per thousand patients, but without supporting facilities, one bed per thousand was actually needed. Adams established a day-hospital program on the St. Pancras psychiatric unit, with places for about 25 patients, but it was not sufficient to handle the number of patients from the catchment area. Adams believes that those institutions which claim that they can care for the population without sending patients on to the mental hospitals are not really telling the whole story. For instance, he stated that a well-known general hospital unit claims to be treating its entire catchment area population of 250,000, although a nearby hostel, operated by a local charitable organization, has been requesting psychiatric nurses to look after the large number of rejects from the hospital. Dr. Adams claimed that these people, who need much supervision, are, in fact, finding unsupervised shelter at the hostel.

Middlesex Hospital maintains a small psychiatric facility at the Woodside Hospital. This is a very well-staffed unit which emphasizes psychotherapy. Middlesex tends to admit patients from all over the country, as is the case for teaching hospitals generally. The Middlesex patients are selected on the basis of their teaching value; no attempt is made to serve Camden in terms of clinical need. University College Hospital found it impractical to try to cater to a population of 120,000 and has reverted to being a little more selective. According to Adams, the psychiatric facilities at University College Hospital have recently been upgraded, but no major changes have yet been made.

Friern Hospital also treats patients on a day basis. These patients come from throughout its catchment area and are former full-time patients who have been returned to the community. It also serves as a night hospital for patients who continue to reside at the hospital but have regular employment in the community. Such patients, who use the hospital more or less as a hostel, are most often those who have no families to return to and for whom no hostel is provided by the local authority.

The patient population of Friern Hospital, because of the areas of London whence they come, are usually quite poor. There are many Negroes and a large number of solitary individuals without home, family, or roots of any kind, who tend to collect in Camden Borough around the railroad stations.

Outpatient clinics, staffed by the consultants from Friern Hospital, operate in a number of areas within Camden Borough. Such clinics are located in the University College Hospital, the Royal Free Hospital, the Whittington Hospital, St. Pancras Hospital, and elsewhere. No outpatient clinic is operated in the Friern Hospital itself.

Friern has eight psychiatric social workers, with various levels of training, who work chiefly with inpatients or their families. Occasionally, they may do case work or group psychotherapy, but they do not participate to any extent in the follow-up of discharged patients. Follow-up is conducted chiefly in the outpatient clinics, since the local-authority social work staff likewise does not follow up patients from the mental hospitals. However, patients discharged from Friern returning to Camden Borough may be referred to the day centers operated by the Camden Local Authority. This is about the full extent of service offered to the hospital by the local authority.

Before the hospital had its own social work staff, the social service staff from Camden Borough's mental health section worked closely with the hospital and tended to be helpful and supportive. However, after the hospital developed its own social work staff, the relationship between the hospital social service department and the social workers of the Camden Borough Local Authority became rather strained. Communication was poor, and there was little cooperation or interaction between the two groups. The social work staff of the Camden Local Authority were repeatedly invited to conferences at the hospital. They attended a few conferences a number of years back but then ceased to show interest. Similarly, the social workers from the mental hospital were invited to attend conferences held by the local authority social work staff but have not done so in recent years.

The relationship between the hospital and the local-authority mental health services has been drastically changed since the implementation of the Seebohm Report. At first, the hospital social workers were attracted by the higher salaries paid by the local authority Social Service Department and initially considered leaving the hospital to work for the local authority. They were reluctant to take the step, however, because they feared a loss of professional identity and were concerned lest they be assigned tasks that were foreign to their own background, experience, and interest. Fortunately, the staff-level social workers at the hospital were given a significant salary increase, putting them nearly in the range of income of the local authority workers at a comparable level. This inducement to keep the workers at the hospital succeeded, and all the psychiatric social workers at Friern elected to stay. In addition, some new PSWs have been added to the hospital staff. These workers gave up better-paying jobs with the local authority to obtain greater job satisfaction at the hospital. With the reorganization of the Health Service, April 1, 1974, following the White Paper, the hospital social workers will be transferred to the Local Authority Social Service Department. The inevitable confusion and additional stress will further intensify the upheaval that followed the Seebohm Report.

Friern is now being used as a clerkship placement for medical students in their next-to-last year of training. The students from University College Hospital are assigned for one week to the outpatient clinics operated at the University College Hospital and spend one day per week for three weeks at the mental hospital itself. Prior to beginning their clinical clerkship at Friern, the students have received no previous training in psychiatry. Recently, a two-month psychiatric clerkship was established, and an increase in time was allotted to didactic teaching and tutorials. The students I met were alert and interested, although somewhat bewildered by what they encountered. They did not give overt evidence of hostility toward psychiatry and seemed interested in learning what they could from their experience. Teaching and research facilities have increased enormously at Friern. The research unit at Friern is now linked with the unit at University College Hospital.

Dr. Adams conducts weekly clinical conferences on each of the wards for which he is responsible. These conferences are attended by the registrar and sister (nurse in charge), and medical students if they are present. The charge nurse on the male ward for the chronically ill seems capable, interested, and dedicated, but his staff is of much more limited capacity. The sister in charge of the female ward for the acutely ill was likewise quite in touch with everything that was going on in her unit. The staff meeting which I attended was attended also by a social worker and an occupational therapist. The level of interest and the vigor of the therapeutic efforts were obviously greater in the acute than in the chronic situation. On the chronic ward even the registrar seemed uninterested in the patients. On the other hand, Adams showed a similar personal investment in both situations. He is obviously a dedicated clinician, working under great handicaps. His dedication is further demonstrated by the manner in which, without support and on his own initiative, and without the knowledge of the hospital authorities, he established the Day Hospital Program on the St. Pancras Psychiatric Unit.

Adams holds a joint appointment with the Camden Local Authority and the University College Hospital and is responsible for the St. Pancras service, which is now officially a part of the University College Hospital. He spends one day per week at Friern and Halliwick Hospitals and one session per week with the social workers in Camden Borough. Part of his Friern time is spent in the outpatient clinics. He spends the rest of his time at St. Pancras and University College Hospitals. Adams is on maximum part time arrangement (9/11) and has two sessions per week for private practice.

As consultant to the local authority, his chief role is to assist the social work staff in planning further community services to meet the needs of the mental patients in Camden. He has often thought that he is unable to stimulate very much activity in this direction and feels that he must wait for the initiative to be taken by the local authority staff. When they seek his advice or guidance, he attempts to influence the directions in which their efforts might go. He seems genuinely interested in strengthening the liaison between the hospital and the local authority staff but feels somewhat at a loss as to how to bring this about. He is not called upon very much by the local-authority staff to function as a clinician.

Adams does not feel that efforts to integrate psychiatry with other medical specialties in the general hospital have been very successful. Most general hospitals still have no programs in psychiatry. When general hospitals do have psychiatric programs, they are usually housed in structures detached from the other hospital facilities. To the observer, it often seems that the hospital authorities and the nonpsychiatric physicians wish to move the psychiatric units as far as possible from the other hospital wards, short of putting them entirely off campus. Adams feels that there may even be some advantage in not having a psychiatric unit as such in a general hospital, so that psychiatric problems will have to be treated on the general wards. He believes that such an approach would force a closer connection between psychiatry and the other specialties. However, he agrees that it is better for the patients to have their own facilities, which are more suited to their particular needs.

Most of the other consultants at Friern have little interest in community work. Nevertheless, the clinical services at Friern will probably be organized along unit lines, each unit to correspond to a particular community catchment area it is to serve. There are some difficulties in bringing this about because of the increased cost in terms of money and staff time that would be involved.

Adams is not certain that community care is, in fact, best for all patients. He believes that a certain number of chronically ill patients are better treated in the hospital than in the community. He is not especially keen on setting up new psychiatric units in general hospitals, because he believes it will require duplication of effort to provide services that can be more economically provided at the mental hospital. On the other hand, he acknowledges that the general hospital units would bring the psychiatric team into closer contact with the patients and make it easier for the patients to receive all-around medical care. He does believe that it is advantageous to have day hospital units in general hospital settings, provided they are not isolated from the other hospital activities.

THE GENERAL PRACTITIONER

There is no system of health teams in Camden Borough, and no social workers are assigned to assist general practitioners in dealing with mental patients. Prior to Seebohm, there were cooperative plans for two general-practitioner groups to establish a health center, with the expectation that social workers would be assigned to it by the local authority mental health section. According to Adams, only a handful of general practitioners in Camden are interested in psychiatric problems, and whenever efforts are made to involve the general practitioners, it is always the same ones who respond. The others seem to try to avoid psychiatric problems. Some are even reluctant to speak directly with the psychiatrist and tend instead to ask the social work staff for advice when confronted by some psychiatric difficulty. Adams believes that this situation reflects the inadequacies of psychiatric teaching in the medical curriculum and represents general attitudes of physicians in community practice. He feels that change will eventually occur as increasing attention is given to psychiatry in medical schools.

VOLUNTARY SERVICES

Primary preventive services in Camden are provided by the Tavistock Centre through its programs of mental health consultation with a variety of care-giving agencies and through direct services offered by the Young Peoples Counselling Service. The Institute for Marital Studies also provides primary preventive services to families. Aside from the programs of the Tavistock, however, the burden of primary prevention is carried by the voluntary agencies in the borough, most specifically the Camden Council of Social Service. This is by far the most important social agency in Camden Borough; the Council and the Camden Association of Mental Health are the two major voluntary organizations providing mental health services in the borough.

The Camden Council of Social Service

The headquarters of the Camden Council of Social Service are located at Kings Cross, opposite the St. Pancras Railroad Station, on the first floor of a building occupied by offices for a number of local-authority and other Camden Borough activities. Along with the administrative offices of the Council of Social Service, the first floor area houses the Citizens' Advice Bureau for that locality.

The Camden Council of Social Service was established December 19, 1964, as an independent voluntary body (92). Its board of directors includes representatives of voluntary organizations and of the statutory authorities in the borough. The council provides machinery for communication and coordination among activities of the voluntary agencies, seeks to discover and fill gaps in service, and provides a number of direct services, including the Citizens' Advice Bureaux, the Department of Social Work, an Adventure Playground, a Voluntary Workers Bureau, and two "clubs." In addition the council publishes a bimonthly newsletter; operates a minibus service, which transports aged and physically disabled clients to various activities; offers inservice training; sponsors an annual borough "Autumn Fair" as a fund-raising venture to benefit local charities; supervises student placements; and informs visitors of local activities. The Camden Council of Social Service is now affiliated with 105 voluntary organizations.

In May 1968, the Camden Borough Council requested that the Camden Council of Social Service review the local charities in the borough and obtain information to help the trustees use their funds to best advantage. Some 80 charities were reviewed and regrouped on an area basis to achieve a more flexible administration.

At the time of my first visit, a very alert and progressive group within the council, under the leadership of Mrs. R. M. Marre, were making a study of their council's activities to anticipate changes in the social service structure as a consequence of the Seebohm Report. Studies included direct services, the constitution of the Council of Social Service, its relationship to the statutory and voluntary agencies, and its fund-raising efforts.

Although the council, itself, does not represent a mental health agency, it is probably· the most important and effective provider of primary preventive mental health services in the borough.

The Citizens' Advice Bureaux (CAB)

The Council operates five CABs on a regular basis which respond to approximately 35,000 calls per year. The bureaux are located at West Hampstead, East Hampstead, Kings Cross, Kentish Town, and Swiss Cottage. The Kings Cross bureau is the busiest, the one at Swiss Cottage the least active. They operate on a five-day week, except at Kentish Town and Swiss Cottage, where offices are open on Saturday mornings as well. The largest number of inquiries regard housing, property, and land. In the Kings Cross and Kentish Town bureaux, family and personal problems likewise provide a large number of callers, while in the East Hampstead bureau, civic, local, and national information is requested by a large proportion of the callers. Other areas of inquiry include employment, consumer trade and manufacture information, questions on social security, health matters, education and training, communication and travel, taxes and duties, and private insurance.

Even before the Seebohm Report, the Camden CAB had decided to experiment by offering a more direct information service to especially vulnerable groups of people. The first such project was a "mini-bureau" set up in a block of new flats called Dorney Towers. This is a public housing project to accommodate people who were formerly living in run-down buildings scheduled for demolition as part of an urban renewal program. The experimental service operated during April 1968, as a result of which the staff became acquainted with the problems facing families or the aged who are forced to move from familiar (though decrepit) surroundings into new, modern high blocks of flats (high-rise apartment buildings). In spite of instructions, some did not understand the need for signing electricity contracts or of informing the board that they had moved in. Old people were literally bewildered by the move, often losing their way. There were problems with pensions and rent payments. The bureau also tried to set up a community action effort, to include a babysitting service and a system of visitors for the aged. The latter efforts failed, because the bureau was unable to put the tenants sufficiently in touch with each other before they had coped with the problems of settling in.

As a result of the Dorney Project, the Camden Borough Council asked the Council of Social Service to undertake another experiment in setting up a neighborhood action group. The goal was to help people become more involved in community decision-making and to work together to meet their own needs.

A second project provided aftercare in the community for prisoners and their families. The clients were male, under 25, and single. The CAB established a liaison with the probation service, the police, and court officials including the magistrates. They attended court sessions and interviewed many prisoners. They found that fewer prisoners lived in Camden than had been anticipated and concluded that a full-time CAB worker at court was unnecessary.

A third project involved an effort at bridging gaps in the statutory legal aid and advice services. The CAB set up an advice panel of volunteer solicitors (lawyers) to whom clients were referred. In one month at the Kings Cross Bureau 12% of the callers at the CAB (68 clients) were referred to the solicitors. If litigation was indicated, the client had to be referred to another solicitor to apply for legal aid. The Holborn Law Society sent volunteers to two other CAB offices (West Hampstead and Kentish Town) for evening consultations. The legal aid program helps people from poor areas to establish contact with solicitors from central London. The clients seem satisfied, and even the CAB workers are impressed with the service offered. A voluntary liaison officer appointed by the Holborn Law Society was chiefly responsible for the success of this project.

A fourth project involved the Greek-speaking Cypriot population in Kentish Town. The CAB had employed a Greek-speaking interpreter on a weekly basis but found this arrangement to be inadequate. The needs of the Cypriot families required a trained Greek-speaking social worker. Fortunately, they found a young Greek married woman who had done casework in the past, and hired her with the help of grants from several private funds. The worker was supervised by the Department of Social Work and dealt with almost 80 Cypriot families. In addition, she ran an evening group for 14 teen-age Cypriot girls.

The Swiss Cottage Bureau established a bereavement service, in cooperation with Dr. C. Murray Parkes of the Tavistock Centre, partly to help with the many practical problems arising at the time of bereavement and partly to serve as an understanding listener for the bereaved. Care was taken to avoid invasion of privacy, and only those who requested help were approached.

In addition to operating the CABs, the Council of Social Service conducts other activities that contribute to the maintenance of mental health.

The Crossways Club

This is a club for city workers over the age of 30, which meets for lunch on Thursday at the Friendship Centre of the Bloomsbury Central Baptist Church. The average age is between 40 and 50. There are 200 members, who welcome the opportunity to make friends and hear talks and discussions. It is operated by a team of volunteers who participate in catering the lunches (average attendance of 60) and in planning and conducting the programs and meetings. The members all work in or near the Holborn area.

Department of Social Work

This small department has been operating a counseling service since 1965 to assist families or individuals with personal problems. Its clients often go first to another source for help, perhaps to a doctor because of insomnia, or to a solicitor for help in ending an intolerable marriage. Many are in the 20 to 28 age group and complain that they feel utterly confused and unable to cope with life. The program serves almost 300 people on a casework basis. Some receive only short-term contact, others continue to be seen regularly over a period of months. The activity responds to a much-felt need in Camden.

The department also supervises social work students from the Stevenage College of Further Education and Chiswick Polytechnic. It has operated a pilot training course for volunteers willing to befriend the families of Camden men or women in prison. After completing the course, the prison visitors were supported by regular group consultations.

The department staff are also available to the constituent organizations of the Camden Council of Social Service in a consultative capacity. Group consultation is also offered to volunteer workers engaged in community work.

Voluntary Workers Bureau

The Voluntary Workers Bureau serves to screen and select volunteers from among many applicants for a variety of assignments. During the 1969–70 year, there were 572 such applicants. The bureau avoids mass recruitment campaigns. They conduct one-day consultation programs on the use of voluntary workers in the social services, in which representatives from over 120 organizations take part. The bureau has referred volunteers for regular work in 56 organizations, in addition to filling about 30 emergency jobs. In addition, the bureau staff have served as advisors to many other Councils of Social Service on setting up a voluntary workers bureau.

The bureau sponsored six one-day seminars during 1968–69 to train volunteers. Ten volunteers were selected to attend a second course, run in cooperation with the Department of Social Work, for those willing to work with ex-prisoners. The number of organizations requesting volunteers continues to grow.

Volunteers do such jobs as mending children's toys, serving as relief helpers for a Children's Department housemother, giving English lessons, doing household tasks, working with mentally retarded children, befriending the handicapped, serving as guides, working with house-bound people, serving lunches at an aged peoples' welfare center, coaching youngsters for their "0" level examinations, and working with families of mental patients.

Parkhill Adventure Playground

This is an activity for underprivileged children between 5 and 16 years of age. Approximately 150 children attended regularly, and during the summer holidays over 230 have attended. The program provides "rugged friendship" as well as a variety of activities. Outings are made to points of interest; football and netball matches on the playground are sponsored in competition with visiting teams. This successful program is not identified as having the preventive mental health function which it so admirably serves.

Pre-Retirement Courses

A unique activity is the provision of information about preparing for retirement. The Council has distributed relevant material to many local firms and organizations; has held several whole-day conferences for personnel and welfare officers on problems of retirement; and, with the help of the Stanhope Institute of Adult Education, has conducted courses for those about to retire. The pre-retirement course includes factual information on pensions, taxes, housing, health and welfare services, use of leisure time, developing hobbies as an active source of employment, and problems of personal adjustment to a new way of life. The courses also help to introduce those about to retire to other services provided by the Camden Council of Social Service.

Recently, the Council of Social Services held an "old students' reunion" for members of the six pre-retirement courses held since 1968 to find out how they were getting along and if the courses had been helpful. Most of them had experienced no major difficulties adjusting to their retirement and thoroughly enjoyed having unlimited free time. However, they were all concerned about inflation and found transportation fares a considerable item in their budgets and rather inhibiting to their activities. Some also felt that there was a subtle difference in the way they were treated by others.

Special Projects

Working groups in behalf of the physically disabled have been organized by the Council of Social Service and include representatives of organizations and individuals interested in trying to make life easier for the physically disabled. They have explored providing transportation through the use of the minibus, problems of employment, and leisure activities. They attempted to prepare a guide book for the disabled, but it was not very successful because of a shortage of necessary volunteers.

Other working groups have functioned in the areas of prison aftercare, housing, voluntary organizations, the needs of young Irish immigrants, and community development.

The Helping Hand Club

The Helping Hand Club, sponsored by the Council of Social Services, is a social organization for former mental patients, which meets on Wednesday afternoons at the council's Euston Road headquarters at Kings Cross. Meetings are conducted by an experienced psychiatric social worker with the assistance of voluntary helpers. Good liaison is maintained with the Kings Cross Citizens' Advice Bureau and the Department of Social Work. The club has made several outings, but the major activity is socializing. The psychiatric social worker and the voluntary staff have made numerous home and hospital visits to help support the members through difficult times.

"Wingfield"

Wingfield Trust, a voluntary organization, brings social and therapeutic help to handicapped children at no cost to their parents. Wingfield began when a group of such children were taught to play old musical instruments, with the idea that the activity would help combat their particular affliction and lessen their isolation. This program has been found particularly beneficial for spastics, severe muscular cases, amputees, and wheelchair victims.

Somers Town

At the request of the Somers Town Study Group, an emergency summer holiday play scheme was developed in an impoverished area with 1,400 children and a shortage of places to play. Local children and young volunteers cleared an area of land of rubble from demolished houses. Funds were donated by various agencies to hire play leaders. Mothers of the children began to offer their help, and more volunteers from the Health Department gave their support. Activities include football games, a Friday night barbecue, a summer youth club, and an under-7 play group. This program has important implications for providing preventive community mental health services and could be emulated in many inner-city situations in the United States.

The Camden Association of Mental Health

The Camden Association of Mental Health, a local chapter of the National Association of Mental Health, is a voluntary group of citizens interested in supporting the community mental health efforts. On their own initiative they managed to raise money and to obtain the support of the local authority, which paid the rental for a hall, called "The Inverness Club," that constitutes their headquarters, and which the association has decorated. Located in a run-down part of Camden Town, the building is unmarked from the outside and therefore quite difficult for the uninitiated to find. It consists mainly of one very large room, furnished with a piano, record player, ping-pong table, and some chairs.

The Monday evening group, which meets at 6:30 P.M., is a "dance and movement" activity, intended to help those without verbal skills to express themselves through physical movement. It is led by two volunteer social workers, who stated that their objective is to "let the patients move according to their own ability." They indicated that some of the activity consisted of dance, some of mime. The principles of psycho-drama were adopted, but not the name, because of a concern that the term "psycho-drama" might be misunderstood. One of the group leaders said that this group activity provided a physical "vocabulary of expression for communication."

The movement-and-dance group was a relatively recent activity of the Mental Health Association, and its nucleus thus far had consisted only of "normal" people, many of whom had been engaged together in this type of activity for some time. They were now trying to attract former patients as members. When asked how the group should be described in order to attract such members and whether the term "dance therapy group" was appropriate, the leader suggested, "Drop the term therapy!"

On Tuesday evening the hall is let to the Royal Free Hospital, who bring their own patient group at 8:00 P.M. for a social evening. It is attended by psychiatric inpatients and outpatients of the hospital.

The best way to convey the scope of the association's activities and manner of operating is to describe one of its meetings. The meeting I observed was well attended, and the participants were enthusiastic. Many were social workers, already involved in their jobs in one or another aspect of mental health service. There were also some people from the local authority, a representative from a labor union, and several psychiatrists. The association operates group activities for former mental patients, and these activities were reviewed at the meeting.

One of the conveners of the meeting stated that she would like to start a discussion group for mothers. She received support from the representative of the Local Authority Children's Department who was present and then asked for volunteers to help run the group. Since the time of the group was tentatively set for 11 A.M. on Wednesdays, the social workers from the Children's Department who were present intimated that, while they might be interested in participating, they would not readily be able to do so during the daytime hours, since they were working.

During the course of the discussion, one of the social workers inquired about the possibility of establishing a group for aged people. Someone replied that most of the members of the "Helping Hand Club" are old people, although it wasn't the purpose of that club to serve aged people specifically. (The Helping Hand Club includes former mental patients not fully recovered who have problems in social interaction.)

The social worker was not satisfied that the Helping Hand Club would answer the need she had in mind. "I had in mind more what you plan for the mothers, a discussion group to examine the problems of the old people, such as they might have in relation to their children." The worker was asked the logical question, "Would you like to run such a group?" She replied that she did not feel skilled enough. But now the possibility of starting a group for the aged gained support, as more and more of the people in attendance became interested and participated in the discussion. I was impressed by the amount of time they spent trying to find a satisfactory leader. Someone indicated that it was also important to have volunteers to drive the old people to the meeting hall and return them to their homes.

Someone suggested that the group should consider the problems of the widowed who had been pushed on to one of the family. "The elderly person likes his independence and does not wish to give up any of it." Another problem was indicated, "Some old people are worried sick about the new decimal system. If this problem could be talked over, it would cease to be a problem." Finally, several volunteers came forth and offered to help organize and operate the group for old people. The emphasis on discussion rather than on socializing was restated. Discussion followed, about the necessity of providing transportation for the aged. Some at the meeting who are themselves over 60 years of age felt that because they managed to get about freely it would be less necessary than some imagined to provide transportation. Others, who had experience in working with the aged, insisted that it was important to have such transportation available even for short distances, otherwise the group would fail. Finally, a retired psychiatrist and the social worker who originally suggested the idea agreed to run the group together. Another social worker also volunteered to help if the group were scheduled for Tuesday afternoon. This seemed a suitable time, and soon others volunteered. Someone suggested that they enlist the aid of Camden Town's Old Peoples' Welfare Department.

The spokesman for the Trade Union Council congratulated the group on their efforts and asked what the council might do to further this one. He described various activities of the trade unions in assisting their membership, including their aged members.

A young priest with a decided brogue spoke up, stating that he had come in order to try to set up something "for Irish unstable boys from Camden Borough." He was interested in any groups for young people which might be formed and agreed to participate in operating a group once it got started. Someone mentioned the Wednesday sessions for young people already being held at Raydon Centre. The social worker who operates the youth group at Raydon Centre asked if it would be possible to transfer that group from the center to the Inverness Club. "We want to inject a community element into the club, and the volunteer group would help to do this. These patients have no friends and we want to help them to make friends." The current president of the Camden Association for Mental Health gave her approval to the transfer on the spot.

There was a call for volunteers for a Wednesday evening group to begin in the fall, and at once someone responded. It was pointed out that each of the groups would need its own secretary, its own coffee-maker, its own "tidy-upper," and a liaison with the Executive Committee of the Mental Health Association. Since the association was involved on Thursdays with a "therapeutic community" (a self-governing patients' group, very unstructured and informal), and since no activities were currently being conducted Fridays, discussion moved to the weekend. Someone said he wanted to start a Sunday lunch club for former mental patients. He asked for two or three volunteers to help for a six- or seven-week period to get the program started. The patients themselves would do the marketing, the cooking, and the cleaning up. Again, there was an immediate and generous response.

The meeting concluded with tea and cookies, but even the social period was spent in further discussion of the programs of the association. I was tremendously impressed by the enthusiasm and dedication of this volunteer group, many of whom worked in the field but were so ready to give freely of themselves in behalf of their patients during their off-duty hours.

afterword

The community mental health program at the crossroads

As this is being written, it has been 14 years since Britain has shifted emphasis in the treatment of the mentally ill from the hospital to the community. During this period many programs involving the mental hospitals and, to some extent, the local authority services have developed. Already, marked changes in social services in Great Britain have followed effectuation of the Seebohm Report (101). A recently reported study of medical education in Britain is bound to have an effect upon medical education in the future (57). The Redcliffe-Maud Report anticipates extensive modifications of local authority services as part of a general reorganization of local government (58). A plan to reorganize the National Health Service, the White Paper, seeks to eliminate the awkward tripartite structure and to create a more unified health care program, regionally organized to correspond to and serve the same areas for which the new local authorities are providing personal and social services (59). Both the local government and the Health Service reorganizations are scheduled for implementation on April 1, 1974.

The general attitude of the medical profession toward the health services continues to be fairly positive, although critical of some facets of its operation. Since current plans to reorganize the National Health Service will affect patterns of delivery of psychiatric services in many ways yet to be determined, it is difficult to predict the future course of community mental health programs in Britain. Nevertheless, certain comments can be made about the service as it has developed thus far and the directions in which it seems to be headed.

Because community mental health services developed with no overall program for coordination or integration of services, and because the structure of the National Health Service was tripartite, the systems which have been established have been severely handicapped in providing continuity of care. Those programs that have managed some degree of continuity of care have done so in spite of these handicaps and represent the efforts of individuals to overcome structural and organizational hindrances of the system within which they must operate. Although the Ministry of Health has repeatedly emphasized that the mental hospital is but one segment of a comprehensive approach to the treatment of the mentally ill, a division of responsibility has remained between the mental hospital services and those developed within the community itself. This division is, to some extent, perpetuated by the White Paper (59), despite its avowed goal of unification of services.

The unique, original efforts that I saw to establish continuity of care (many of which were later emulated by others) fell into one of three categories. First, services provided by the mental hospitals were essentially an extension into the community of in-hospital programs, using the manpower of the hospital staff to operate clinics or day treatment programs, such as the program at Graylingwell Hospital in Chichester. Second, services developed by the local authority, usually with the strong support of the MOH, used the psychiatric social work staff of the mental health section of the health department to operate day centers, sheltered workshops, or other community programs, as exemplified by the Camden Borough services. Third were efforts at true collaboration and joint participation of the staffs of the mental hospitals with the resources and manpower of the Local Authority Health Department, an outstanding example of which is found at Croydon.

Paradoxically, the creation of the new unified Social Service Department, which was intended to improve the quality and continuity of personal social services, had the effect of damaging severely those community mental health programs operated chiefly by the psychiatric social workers of the local authority. The disruptions precipitated by Seebohm provoked attempts to circumvent its effects, such as the appointment in Newham of the former MOH, Dr. Dennison, to be Director of the new Social Services Department, or attempts there and elsewhere to continue to give social workers task assignments on a disciplinary, categorical basis rather than according to the generic concept prescribed by Seebohm.

It is clear that matters will not remain as they now are, and many former patterns of providing continuity of care will undergo change. As the locus of hospital care for the mentally ill shifts from mental institutions to district general hospitals (in effect, to the community), there will be a corresponding alteration in the organization of community services now provided by the mental hospitals. Possibly the least disorganization will occur where strong collaborative working relationships exist, as in Croydon, and where there already are strong general hospital services, such as in the Manchester Region (Blackburn and Salford).

It appears to me that the structural changes in the offing will bring the British pattern of community mental health service closer to its American counterpart. I believe that although this will necessitate the sacrifice of some excellent existing patterns of care, the overall result will be marked facilitation of continuity of care and integration of effort.

Local authorities have remained laggard in assuming responsibility for providing community-based treatment for the mentally ill and continue to provide only minimal service. Disparities among the services provided by different local authorities are glaring, and no consistent national program of community mental health can be developed in the face of such uneven provisions. At times the local authorities have moved in to fill vacuums left by mental hospitals which have failed to carry out their end of the program, but at other times such vacuums have merely remained. The local authorities have consistently expended more on behalf of the mentally retarded than the mentally ill, and their future plans call for a continuance of that tendency. Furthermore, the responsibilities of the local authorities for providing other community services have tended to take priority with regard to their interest, attention, and resources.

Where services are provided, it has not always been clear which responsibilities properly belong to local authority and which to the mental hospital. Plans for local government reorganization and for the reorganization of the health service do not significantly change the distribution of responsibility for providing community mental health services. However, I believe that two factors will greatly influence the manner in which these services are actually provided in practice: the creation of the Social Service Department and the emphasis upon the district general hospitals as major providers of psychiatric services.

The generic orientation of the Social Service Department will, I believe, tend to weaken the programs in those communities which have pursued the development of mental health facilities most aggressively and imaginatively. In those communities the PSWs were the best-trained social workers in the local authority and constituted an elite corps often resented by other social workers. With the formation of the new Social Service Department, PSWs were outnumbered by other workers, and at the same time, were stripped of their elite status by being tossed into the same generic hopper with their trained, partly trained, and untrained colleagues from the Welfare Department and the Children's Department.

Another consequence of Seebohm (101) has been to strip the MOH of many of his responsibilities, a predicament not remedied by the

White Paper (59). Thus the MOH, previously a prime agent in motivating the local authority to support mental health programs in those instances where the local authority had developed strong services, is no longer a viable spokesman for the cause of mental health in the chambers of local government. (An interesting exception is found in Newham, where the MOH, Dr. Dennison, was appointed Director of the new Social Service Department.)

On the other hand, the arrival on the community scene of a cadre of psychiatric personnel to man the newly developing general hospital programs will tend to increase the psychiatrist's involvement in community mental health activities. I believe this will especially be true where the retrenchment of local authority services subsequent to Seebohm has created a new vacuum. To be sure, certain psychiatrists will continue to regard their province as the institution rather than the community and will conduct the general hospital psychiatric unit as if it were merely the old mental hospital moved to a new location. Since many institutional programs have already developed some community involvement, however, it is difficult to imagine that most psychiatrists based at general hospitals will be unresponsive to community needs.

I believe that these psychiatrists will turn their attention increasingly to the more acute aspects of mental illness and will become involved in early intervention and intensive short-term treatment. I expect that they will continue to follow their post-hospital patients in the clinics, dispense medications, and remain alert for the return of symptoms (such as has been the pattern at St. Mary Abbots Hospital). I think they will have neither the resources nor the inclination, however, to become involved in retraining and resocialization programs, let alone the operation of special living accommodations, such as hostels or half-way houses.

I expect that psychiatrists will be very much aware of the need for such services, however, and will turn to the Social Service Department to see that these needs are met. Thus, they will provide the stimulus which previously had come from the MOH (in those communities where local authorities developed strong programs) but with even greater intensity. I believe the Social Service Departments, in most instances, will be responsive to these expressions. Social workers like to be helpful; if additional resources have to be extracted from the local government, social workers will be motivated to press for them, as it will be their own empire rather than someone else's that will be enhanced thereby.

To sum up, I believe that local authority activity in community mental health programs will initially be reduced, while psychiatrists at district general hospitals will take a more active role. In time, the new Social Service Department will pressure local authorities to provide facilities and resources to a much greater extent than in the past. I also foresee the development in many communities of a viable collaborative arrangement between the General Hospital Psychiatry Department and the Social Service Department.

The incumbent psychiatric leadership in the Health Ministry is committed to the strategy of basing major inpatient programs for the mentally ill in district general hospitals (42). An inevitable corollary of this trend is a sharp constriction of the role of large free-standing mental institutions. It is unlikely that the mental hospitals will be phased out altogether, as had initially been anticipated in some quarters; the "deteriorated" long-term patient, unable to function without continuous care and supervision, as well as the growing, so-called psycho-geriatric population, still an unresolved problem, will most likely be dealt with by existing facilities and staffs of the mental hospitals. In the future, the majority of new cases and the younger mentally ill population will probably never see the inside of these traditional institutions.

Dr. A. A. Baker, major architect and spokesman for the policy of reliance on general-hospital psychiatric departments, has himself had personal experience with the effectiveness and potential of such units (2). The purpose-built unit he established at St. Mary Abbots Hospital in London has managed the many acute and emergency problems thrust upon it, and at the same time has utilized outpatient and day hospital facilities, in addition to its inpatient capacity, to avoid institutionalizing many of its patients. I expect that, despite some voices of protest or attacks from the press (87), the mental health effort will continue to be concentrated upon the general hospitals.

Emphasis upon the general hospital will of course have multiple consequences for the entire community mental health program at a number of levels. First, basing the psychiatrist in the community rather than at some outlying institution will bring him into more immediate proximity with the programs and problems in the community, and will alter basic patterns of psychiatric practice; psychiatry will become more community-oriented and less hospital-oriented. I expect that the majority of mental health problems in the community, particularly acute cases, will increasingly be dealt with by psychiatrists as medical-psychiatric problems rather than being regarded as social service problems. Psychiatrists will give greater emphasis to prevention, with the development of crisis-intervention services and perhaps, some efforts at early case-finding. Therapeutic intervention is likely to become more prompt and more intensive, while length of in-hospital stay will continue to decrease. Day hospital programs will, I believe, become integral components of general hospital psychiatric services, and ambulatory services (already widely available) will receive greater emphasis as an alternative to hospitalization. I foresee the clinics being used for managing outpatients who have never been hospitalized, using psychotherapy in addition to the more traditional modalities.

An American psychiatrist must keep in mind that, for the most part, what he understands as psychotherapy is quite foreign to most of his British counterparts. Many British psychiatrists are still suspicious of psychotherapy as we know it, if not openly hostile to it. What the average British psychiatrist means when he says that he uses psychotherapy is that he spends a few moments to chat with his patient, gives him some words of encouragement or a pat on the back, and sets up a return appointment. It is difficult for the average British psychiatrist who has not visited the United States to conceptualize how psychotherapy, as we know it, fits into the scheme of care for the psychotic, pre-psychotic, or borderline patient. Only a few months ago I received an inquiry from an important British study group examining architectural requirements for psychiatric units, as to whether it was necessary to include facilities for group therapy in the design. I expect, however, that there will be experiential as well as educational changes which will make these approaches more familiar to our British colleagues, that these changes will lead to a reassessment of the value of the method, and that this reassessment will be reflected, in turn, in an increased utilization of psychotherapy for individuals, groups, and families.

On the other hand, I believe that rehabilitative programs (particularly those involving reduction of disability, retraining, resocialization, and the provision of half-way houses, hostels, and other living accommodations) will remain under the aegis of the Social Service Department. I would hope that social workers will become rather frequent visitors to the clinics of general hospital units to become acquainted with the patients and to consult with the psychiatrists.

A net effect of the focus on general hospital psychiatry will be, I believe, to enhance continuity of care and to shift the emphasis toward preventive efforts, crisis intervention, prompt and intensive treatment, and shorter periods of hospitalization. The British will accustom themselves to the "revolving door" and will recognize, as we have in the United States, that several short in-hospital periods are preferable to a single long one, in terms of economy as well as reduction of the consequences of institutionalism.

Basing mental health care at general hospitals will most likely bring the psychiatrist into closer proximity with his other medical colleagues, although one cannot assume that this will definitely be the case. Psychiatric units, as they exist today in the general hospitals in England, continue to be rather isolated from other hospital facilities and activities, and there is little professional exchange between psychiatrists and other physicians. To some extent this reflects a mutual wish for separation. Many psychiatrists are still quite insecure and defensive about their medical identity, while many physicians who are not in psychiatry continue to hold the speciality in low esteem and regard psychiatrists as medical misfits.

As psychiatry continues to upgrade standards of education and performance, and as its enhanced status in consequence of the charter of the Royal College of Psychiatrists becomes more apparent, psychiatrists are bound to lose some of their self-consciousness and will begin to offer their services to other areas of the hospital. If this occurs, I am certain that there will be a gradual rise, however grudging, in the stature of psychiatry in the eyes of the medical profession. As psychiatry demonstrates its relevance, it will be called upon more frequently. Since emotional complications often accompany somatic illness, patients from elsewhere in the hospital may be transferred (temporarily) to the psychiatric unit, requiring internists or surgeons to set foot in this now alien province. This will provide the psychiatrist and his medical colleagues a chance to know each other better.

There are many problems still to be worked out. The new administrative structure of the Health Service will alter existing relationships with the agencies responsible for the distribution of resources. Furthermore, the psychiatrist at the general hospital will be a spokesman for a mere department rather than for an entire institution. Those who remember the history of the distribution of "Distinction Awards" among the specialties fear that psychiatry at the general hospital is liable to come out at the short end (87). I am sanguine about the long range prospects, however. British psychiatry is not lacking in capable leadership and articulate spokesmen.

The general practitioner is not and has not been a part of the overall community mental health effort, because of the tripartite structure of the National Health Service and because of the reluctance of general practitioners themselves to become involved. Most of them tend to avoid patients with problems of mental illness and have not been effective in identifying early cases of such problems. Some have even refused to restore former patients to their rolls, if the patients have spent a long time at a mental hospital. Others have been less negative, but their participation has been limited, for the most part, to regulating medications following the patient's discharge from the hospital. A few have expressed interest in psychiatry and have attended the special courses offered by the Tavistock and other institutions, but it has been difficult for them to utilize their new knowledge because of time and other pressures.

The American reader must keep in mind that while psychiatry has become an increasingly important part of the medical school curriculum in the United States over the past two decades, it has only recently been introduced as a distinct program of instruction in some medical schools in England. Even in those medical schools whose curriculum has included psychiatry for a long time, the emphasis has been minor, so that the educational background of the average British general practitioner has been limited in psychiatry.

In addition to his unfamiliarity with psychiatric precepts and practice, the general practitioner often shares the anti-psychiatric prejudices of his non-psychiatric specialist colleagues, although perhaps to a lesser extent. The average general practitioner is certainly aware that the majority of his patients present emotional symptoms along with their somatic complaints and that some of their somatic symptomatology is entirely emotional in origin, but he is not likely to think of the psychiatrist in connection with these problems. British psychiatry has had little to do with psychoneurotic or psychosomatic disorders; it has been concerned almost exclusively with chronic mental illnesses, usually psychotic in nature, and usually after the patient has been admitted to the mental hospital. General practitioners thus have called upon the psychiatrist only when their patient was sick enough to require hospitalization.

Several factors are likely to change this state of affairs in the future. Changes in medical education in the wake of the Todd Report will give new emphasis to psychiatry in the medical school curriculum (57). Greater emphasis will probably be given to psychodynamics, personality development, and emotional aspects of physical illness as well. Thus, newly graduating physicians will be much more psychiatrically sophisticated than their predecessors. Further, the trend toward establishing "health teams," already evident in some areas such as Salford, will bring the general practitioner into a closer working relationship with the local authority staff, particularly social workers and health visitors. This arrangement will provide the general practitioner contact with other professionals with whom he can share the burdens of the emotional problems presented by his patients. These factors should combine to make the general practitioner of the future more aware of and sensitive to the emotional needs of his patients, more attentive to the emotional aspects of their illnesses, and better able to identify psychiatric illnesses earlier in their course.

It is also likely that the development of psychiatric services in district general hospitals will make it easier for the general practitioner to refer patients for evaluation and treatment before the patient's psychiatric illness reaches crisis or major psychotic proportions. Hopefully psychiatrists will come to recognize the value of early intervention in bringing about prompt functional improvement and in avoiding, in many instances, the problems of chronic disablement. In that event, psychiatric clinics at the district general hospitals would carry a significant case load of ambulatory patients who have never been hospitalized, in contrast to the present situation where most clinic cases are former inpatients.

Increasing psychiatric sophistication on the part of general practitioners, including greater sensitivity to early manifestations of psychiatric disorders, coupled with more readily available resources for referral, should facilitate early case-finding and prompt psychiatric intervention, provided the psychiatrists themselves become attuned to the value of vigorous early treatment in forestalling the debilitating consequences of long-term institutionalization. While general practitioners may thus be expected to make more frequent psychiatric referrals of patients with milder manifestations of psychopathology, it is unlikely that they will themselves take a more active therapeutic role with these patients.

One of the most glaring difficulties in establishing comprehensive community mental health service in Britain is the disorganization of psychiatric services for children. Services for "disturbed children," such as they are, are provided via child guidance clinics and special schools run by the Local Authority Education Department. The Medical Officer of Health has usually been the chief medical officer for the Education Department, and these services have usually had the support, if not the active guidance, of child psychiatrists. Because of the volume of work, however, the actual "treatment" of children, particularly those with behavioral disorders, learning problems, situational maladjustments, and neurotic and personality difficulties, has been carried out by teachers and educational psychologists rather than by the child psychiatrist, who acts only as a consultant, gives advice, or provides supervision.

In addition, services for "maladjusted children" are distinct from services for "autistic children," who are put into a completely separate category. The local authority does not provide ambulatory services for autistic children, and there are very few hospitals for them. The day program for autistic children operated by the Marlborough Day Hospital is a rare program. Other hospitals for mentally ill children, such as the Great Ormond Street Children's Hospital and the Maudsley Hospital, are likewise few and far between.

Physician-operated clinics for children are relatively uncommon. As I observed, in both the Tavistock and the Institute of Family Psychiatry in Ipswich, children's services are linked to those for parents or families.

The integration of children's psychiatric services ("Child Guidance Service") and the community mental health service of the Local Authority Health Department, such as I observed in the London borough of Newham, is rare. The child-psychiatry background of Dr. Kahn, psychiatrist in charge of the mental health program in the Local Authority Health Department, doubtless accounts for Newham's integrated program.

Today services for emotionally disturbed children are still quite fragmented. Such children may be treated in child guidance clinics operated by the local authorities and staffed by educational psychologists and social workers; in so-called "joint clinics" in which a health service psychiatrist augments the local authority staff, usually on local authority premises; or in child psychiatric clinics, which are based chiefly in general hospitals and are operated by the health service. The latter, which have the best trained psychiatrists and all of the training posts in child psychiatry, also operate the only inpatient facilities for emotionally disturbed children.

Psychiatrists have long recognized that mental health services for children are properly a medical responsibility. Following the reorganization of the National Health Service, all psychiatric services for children will became the responsibility of the Health Service. Furthermore, the Royal Medico-Psychological Association has recommended dropping the term "child guidance" in favor of "child psychiatric clinics," to further emphasize this recognition. The latter term is already receiving increasing usage.

A 1973 discussion paper from the Health Ministry (122) recommends that child psychiatric services be developed as part of the district general hospital services and that they establish links with the school psychological services, child health services, and the social services department. These services are expected to be manned by a multi-disciplinary team consisting of child psychiatrists, psychologists, nurses, social workers, teachers, doctors in related specialities, and other workers.

The paper recommends that child psychiatric services be organized on a health area basis in order to make the most effective use of the limited number of child psychiatrists and to provide an optimal size for a child psychiatric unit. The bed requirement of such an inpatient unit is estimated to be 20 beds per million population. An optimum-sized inpatient unit of 15 beds is expected to serve a total population of from 500,000 to 1,200,000. This means that child psychiatric inpatient services would not be available to each health district but would be concentrated into one or two units within a health area, depending on the size of that area and its population.

To meet existing childrens' mental health needs, a ratio of one consultant child psychiatrist to a population of 50,000 children under the age of 16 is suggested. This is equivalent to one consultant to a total population of 200,000. Since the average health district is likely to have a population of 250,000, the area makes a more suitable basis for organization than the smaller district.

The present national average ratio of consultant child psychiatrists to total population is 1:250,000, with considerable regional variations (from 1:146,000 to 1:600,000). To achieve the recommended ratio of 1:200,000, the number of consultant posts must increase at the rate of 5% per year. Many psychiatrists regard this goal as inadequate and believe that the proposal makes inadequate provisions for other staff as well. An intensive educational effort will be required to provide a sufficient number of child psychiatrists as well as other trained members of the "interdisciplinary team," if the anticipated program is to succeed.

Child psychiatric clinics are expected to provide clinical services primarily for investigating and treating emotionally disturbed children, and to a much lesser extent, mentally ill children. Local education-authorities will continue to furnish educational psychology services in the schools. In view of the shortage of child psychiatrists, a British Psychological Society report has advocated the trebling of educational psychologists to perform the work of the unavailable psychiatrists (68). It would seem more appropriate, however, to increase efforts toward medical training and to produce the required number of child psychiatrists (68).

There are practically no facilities for adolescents, but the Health Ministry has issued guidelines for development of adolescent inpatient units. A circular on adolescent outpatient services will soon be issued by the Health Ministry.

The management of mental retardation problems has been largely the province of the local authorities operating under the Medical Officer of Health through the Mental Health Department. Many local authorities have developed facilities for mentally retarded children, including day schools, training centers, and sheltered living accommodations. Similar provisions have been made for mentally retarded adults, including sheltered workshops and industrial rehabilitation units. Even many of the severely retarded have been maintained in the community. This has been the one area in which the local authority could maintain a coordinated program involving both children and adults but the program may end with the approaching transfer of responsibility to the Education Department.

Physicians have actually shown little real interest in the retardation problem, except where genetic or metabolic factors are involved. The major responsibilities for continuing care of mentally subnormal children and adults have been carried almost exclusively by non-medical personnel, even when the programs were based in the mental health section of the health department. Since Seebohm (101) and the White Paper (59) have effectively dismantled the Local Authority Health Department, it is probable that programs for the mentally subnormal will fare better under the aegis of the Education Department, which has sufficient manpower, organization, and interest to obtain the necessary financial support to sustain and enlarge these programs.

While the reorganization of medical education in the wake of the

Todd Report (57) will undoubtedly increase the emphasis on psychiatry in the medical schools, dangers as well as benefits are to be anticipated. For example, Tetlow (105) warns that bureaucratization of medical education may stifle the development of innovative approaches, and Ellul (22) cautions against the production of technologists rather than well-rounded, humane physicians, a caution echoed with a variety of overtones by Dornhurst and Hunter (21), Hill (63), Platt (90), and Woodmansey (119). Sudden expansion of medical school departments may impair the quality of teaching, and Lawless (76) draws attention to potential difficulties associated with too ready acceptance of the comfort and security afforded by membership in the establishment.

Even where the Todd Report is expected to have a favorable effect on undergraduate medical education, the need to improve postgraduate education remains. Hospitals outside of London still lack formalized educational opportunities; more active teaching and supervision are needed than are presently available. The need for a more effective method of assessing the competence of psychiatrists is widely recognized. The feeling is also widespread that the curriculum content requires modification, although the proposals for change are by no means unanimously favored. It has been urged that greater emphasis be placed on clinical competence and less on the basic sciences, and many have insisted that trainee psychiatrists be equipped with psychotherapeutic skill. One objection is that many trainee psychiatrists without aptitude in this area would remain inept in comparison to other medical or even non-medical colleagues. It has been pointed out that one-to-one psychotherapy can never meet the community mental health problem, an observation which merely brings the retort that this fact emphasizes the need for training in psychotherapy for psychiatrists. There will need to be a large-scale delegation of mental health functions to general practitioners, health visitors, and social workers, the argument runs; and since psychiatrists will be responsible for their training and supervision, the psychiatrists will require skill in psychotherapy to carry out these responsibilities (105).

The new Royal College of Psychiatrists will determine to a great extent the future content and course of psychiatric education. The examination for admission to the college promises to be a factual test based on a rigid medical model, which has brought forth voices of concern and the recommendation that the MRC Psych examination be kept under critical review (105).

Accreditation of training programs, improvement of libraries, and increased availability of audio-visual teaching aids such as videotape systems are needed. Many British psychiatrists and educators, studying the American model of residency-training and board examinations, are pressing for emulation of at least some aspects of the United States system.

It is difficult to foresee the ultimate direction that psychiatric education will take in Britain because of the current differences of opinion within the profession itself. An observer senses a power struggle between those psychiatrists committed to the traditional basic science, neurologically oriented, medical-organic model and those seeking to give greater emphasis to a more dynamic, psychotherapeutic orientation; and the outcome of this struggle, more than any other factor, will determine the education, and hence the professional characteristics, of the British psychiatrist of tomorrow.

Although we have focused our attention on the problems of the British system the American reader should keep in mind that the community mental health services in the United States have numerous problems of their own, many of which are similar to those of the British. Further, it would seem that the British have been much more innovative and better prepared to cope with problems than we have been in the United States. For example, despite the fact that community mental health programs in the United States have developed in a different fashion and have emphasized different aspects than the programs developed in Britain, nevertheless, there has been a comparable tendency in the United States to reduce the state hospital populations by discharge of large numbers of patients into the community. This has often been done without adequate prior preparation of patients for discharge, such as vocational training or resocialization efforts. Patients have been discharged on oral medications even though it is widely recognized that at least 50% of them do not take oral medication regularly (121). There has been no general development of community facilities to receive them such as sheltered living accommodations, nor has there been any effective program for securing employment of former hospital residents. In effect, the burden of responsibility has merely been shifted from the hospitals to the communities; the community mental health centers, in most instances, have not developed adequate facilities or programs for community care of former hospital patients and have been largely neglectful of them. The trend has been criticized by many American psychiatrists who consider that both the patient and the community are less well off than before.

In some areas, Britain is answering simple human needs in ways that we in the United States are not, and we could well borrow ideas and methods from several of their programs. Some of the British models which might be incorporated into the community mental health system in the United States include: the Citizens' Advice Bureaux, hospitals for terminally ill patients, industrial therapy programs, therapeutic social clubs, and direct personal supportive services within the community, such as well-supervised sheltered living accommodations, "meals on wheels," and home helps.

While some of the specific services offered by the Citizens' Advice Bureaux may be similar to those now provided by social agencies such as Family Service societies, there is for the most part no American parallel to the CABs. These voluntary agencies provide a service for anyone with a question or problem. The kinds of service they offer could well be included as part of the community mental health services offered by a community mental health center, in the form of a clinic for the problems of daily living. Such a clinic, while under the auspices of the total mental health program, would not require that its clientele be diagnosed as mentally ill or emotionally disturbed. Rather, people with ordinary problems of coping with the vicissitudes of daily living, those faced by transitional life crises (marriage, raising a family, death of a loved one, etc.), and people struggling with habit difficulties (smoking, overeating, drinking) could seek help at such a clinic. In the United States, certain "storefront" outreach projects do aid the lower socioeconomic groups, but there is nothing comparable for middle-class people. At Sinai Hospital of Detroit we have established a middle-class-oriented Problems of Daily Living Clinic, and I can attest its value.

There is no program in the United States comparable to St. Christopher's Hospice which, although not a mental health service, serves an important and valuable preventive mental health function. In our country, attention to the mental health aspects of death and dying has been a recent development. Today eight out of ten Americans die in hospitals and nursing homes, cut off from friends and relatives, and forced to face death alone (74). St. Christopher's pioneering experiment, designed to relieve the physical, mental, and spiritual distress associated with death, could well serve as a model to be emulated here.

The United States has no program comparable to the British "Meals on Wheels." Volunteers deliver three meals a day (prepared in kitchens operated by the local authority) to aged or handicapped people who are unable to prepare food for themselves. Without this service, these people would have to be cared for in institutions. Not only does "Meals on Wheels" answer a human need, it reduces the demand for hospital beds.

The local authority also provides "home helps," who periodically come into the home and help those temporarily incapacitated and unable to manage a household. The closest parallel we have to this program is the Visiting Nurse Association (VNA), but the amount of service it provides falls short of the home help system. Furthermore, the VNA is geared toward managing patients with acute medical problems rather than those with chronic disabilities, and it is unable usually to provide services for mental patients.

In the United States, industrial therapy programs are geared almost entirely for physically handicapped people. Recently, a few industrial therapy programs have been established for the mentally ill, but most mental institutions provide only occupational therapy. Although occupational therapy helps to restore mental health, it does not prepare the patient for employment in the community or provide him with a job once he gets out of the hospital. The industrial therapy workshops in England offer not only therapy but training in vocational skills, and job placement.

Another program which reflects Britain's emphasis on rehabilitation is the therapeutic social club. The club helps to facilitate resocialization in the community for patients who have just been released from the hospital. For patients who are severely disabled and not prepared to make a complete adjustment to the community, the club may be their only social outlet.

In at least one instance a British program has been introduced into this country. Since 1968 the Richmond Fellowship has begun to establish hostels in the United States. There are no reports yet of the effectiveness of this "transplant," however. The "group homes" program is another innovation that has been tried in the United States, but the setup and management have been different from the British model. The program has been used in the United States with questionable success as part of the rehabilitation program for narcotic addicts. More recently it has been employed for detoxification and rehabilitation of alcoholics.

The major difference in social organization of the two countries makes any comprehensive replication of their system of social services impossible. Since social services in Britain are organized as a governmental function, an otherwise admirable program may be impossible to emulate in our country. While Britain is a "welfare state," committed to providing social and health services for its citizens from the "cradle to the grave," the United States sees itself as a country of self-made citizens. Americans are expected to be independent and self-reliant, and one is frequently looked down upon if he requires assistance from a social agency or charitable organization, and particularly if he is dependent upon government welfare for his support.

As Britain prepares to inaugurate a coordinated regional health care delivery system based on the recommendations of the White Paper, I have ventured to predict some of the consequences of that reorganization. Unquestionably there will be upheavals reminiscent of those that followed implementation of the Seebohm Report. These will, I believe, be transitory, and in the long run, the reorganization will be seen as beneficial.

Ideally, the new scheme would facilitate earlier detection and treatment of psychiatric problems, wider availability and closer coordination of post-hospital care, and greater continuity of care in general. Integration of psychiatric practice into community general hospitals will have a salutory effect on the status of psychiatry and psychiatrists, and it may eventually influence the medical school curriculum and patterns of postgraduate training as well. We may expect improvements in care for children and adolescents by virtue of the consolidation of this responsibility within the Health Service.

It would be hazardous to make detailed predictions about local situations, because as we have already noted, much depends on the imagination and energies of those charged with implementing a particular program. If the past is a reliable guide, however, we have reason to expect that British inventiveness and ingenuity will again rise to the occasion and that psychiatry as a whole will be the better for it.

references*

1. Akhurst, C. R. 1968. Remarks of the editor, The Seebohm Report. Brit. Quarterly J. Social Work, Vol. 25, October.

2. Baker, A. A. 1968. Do we need psychiatric hospitals? In What's wrong with the mental health services? Report of the Annual Conference. London: National Association for Mental Health, pp. 16-22.

3. ———. 1968. Psychiatric nursing in the community. In The treatment of mental disorders in the community. Daniels and Freeman, eds. London: Bailliere, Tindall, and Cassell.

4. Baker, A. A.; Morison, M.; Game, J. A.; and Thorpe, J. G. 1961. Admitting schizophrenic mothers with their babies. Lancet 2: 237-239.

5. Bierer, J. 1951. The day hospital: an experiment in social psychiatry and syntho-analytic psychotherapy. London: H. K. Lewis.

6. British addiction rate drops under M.D. control. 1971. Psychiatric News, Vol. 6, No. 23, pp. 1 and 15.

7. Brook, C. P. B. and Stafford-Clark, D. 1961. Psychiatric treatment in general wards. Lancet 1: 1159.

8. Brooke, E. M. 1962. Factors affecting the demand for psychiatric beds. Lancet 2: 1211.

9. Capoore, H. S. and Nixon, J. W. G. 1961. Short-stay psychiatric unit in a general hospital. Lancet 2: 1531.

10. Carse, J. 1959. The Worthing experiment. London: South West Metropolital Regional Hospital Board.

*Note: Her Majesty's Stationery Office is abbreviated H.M.S.O.
Health Memorandum is abbreviated H.M.

11. ———. 1961. Community care and treatment of the psychiatric patient. The Practitioner 187: 672-678.

12. Carse, J.; Panton, N. E.; and Watt, A. A. 1958. District mental health service: the Worthing experiment. Lancet 1: 39-41.

13. Carstairs, G. M.; Walton, H. J.; Smythies, J. R.; and Crisp, A. H. 1968. Survey of undergraduate psychiatric teaching in the United Kingdom. Brit. J. Psychiat. 114: 1411-1416.

14. Cohen, N. and Haldane, F. 1962. Inpatient psychiatry in general hospitals. Lancet 1: 1113.

15. College of Psychiatry. 1963. Brit. med. J. 2: 1328.

16. Community Mental Health Centers Construction Act. 1963. P. L. 88-164, 77: Stat. 282. From Public Papers of the Presidents, No. 447.

17. Cooper, A. B. and Early, D. F. 1961. Evolution in the mental hospital. Brit. med. J. 1: 1603.

18. Cotton, J. M. 1962. Integrated psychiatric unit in a general hospital: a case history. Trustee. January.

19. Curran, D. 1964. Organized psychiatry. Lancet 1: 1102.

20. Diggory, P.; Peel, J.; and Potts, M. 1970. Preliminary assessment of the 1967 abortion act in practice. Lancet 1: 287-291.

21. Dornhurst, A. C. and Hunter, A. 1967. Fallacies in medical education. Lancet 2: 666-667.

22. Ellul, J. 1965. The technological society. New York: Random House.

23. Enoch, D. M. 1971. The organization of psychogeriatrics. J. G. Howells, ed. London: The Society of Clinical Psychiatrists.

24. Eysenck, H. J. 1969. Relapse and symptom substitution after different types of psychotherapy. Beh. Res. & Ther. 7: 283-287.

25. ———. 1970. Behavior therapy and its critics. J. beh. Ther. & Psychiat. 1: 5-15.

26. Farndale, J. 1961. The day hospital movement in Great Britain. London: Pergamon.

27. Fox, R. 1968. The law on abortion. Lancet 1: 542-543.

28. Freeman, H. 1960. Oldham and district psychiatric service. Lancet 1: 218-221.

29. ———. 1968. Community psychiatry. Brit. J. Psychiat. 114: 481-484.

30. ———. 1968. The structure of the local authority and hospital service in relation to mental health. In The treatment of mental disorders

in the community. Daniels and Freeman, eds. London: Bailliere, Tindall, and Cassell.

31. Furman, Sylvan S. 1965. Community mental health services in northern Europe. Washington, D.C.: Department of Health, Education, and Welfare, No. 1407.

32. Glaser, F. B. and Ball, J. C. 1971. The British narcotic "register" in 1970, a factual review. JAMA 216: 1177-1182.

33. Gordon, Israel. 1969. Seebohm sophistry and green paper gallimaufry. Lancet 1: 299-300.

34. Great Britain. Central Office of Information, Reference Division. 1968. Health services in Britain, pamphlet 20. London: H.M.S.O.

35. ———. Central Office of Information, Reference Division. 1969. Social services in Britain, pamphlet 3, London: H.M.S.O.

36. ———. Department of Health and Social Security, Information Services Division. 1968. National health service notes. London: H.M.S.O.

37. ———. Department of Health and Social Security. 1970. Annual report, 1969. Cmnd. 4462, London: H.M.S.O.

38. ———. Department of Health and Social Security. 1971. Annual report 1970. Cmnd. 4714, London: H.M.S.O.

39. ———. Department of Health and Social Security. 1970. Hospital advisory service's examination of long-stay hospitals. H.M. (70) 17, London: H.M.S.O.

40. ———. Department of Health and Social Security. 1970. National health service: the future of the national health service. London: H.M.S.O.

41. ———. Department of Health and Social Security. 1971. On the state of the public health: annual report of the chief medical officer, 1969. London: H.M.S.O.

42. ———. Department of Health and Social Security. 1971. Hospital services for the mentally ill. H.M. (71) 97, London: H.M.S.O.

43. ———. Department of Health and Social Security. 1972. Report of the working party on medical administrators. H.M.S.O.

44. ———. Digest of health statistics for England and Wales. 1971. London: H.M.S.O.

45. ———. Journal Department of the British Medical Association. 1972. The mental health service after unification–report of the Tripartite Committee. London: H.M.S.O.

46. ———. Labor Party. 1946. National Health Service Act. Citation 9 and 10, George 6, Chap. 81.

47. ———. Ministry of Education. 1948. Circular 179. London: H.M.S.O.

48. ———. Ministry of Education. 1955. Report of the committee on maladjusted children. London: H.M.S.O.

49. ———. Ministry of Health. 1947. Memorandum, R.H.B. 47 (13). London: H.M.S.O.

50. ———. Ministry of Health. 1962. A hospital plan for England and Wales. Cmnd. 1604. London: H.M.S.O.

51. ———. Ministry of Health. 1963. Health and welfare: the development of community care. London: H.M.S.O.

52. ———. Ministry of Health. 1966. The hospital building programme: a revision of the hospital plan for England and Wales. Cmnd. 3000. London: H.M.S.O.

53. ———. Ministry of Health. 1967. Annual report for the year 1967. Cmnd. 3702. London: H.M.S.O.

54. ———. Ministry of Health and Department of Health for Scotland. 1961. Joint working party on the medical staffing structure in the hospital service report. London: H.M.S.O.

55. ———. Review Body on Doctors' and Dentists' Remuneration. 1969. Tenth report. London: H.M.S.O.

56. ———. Royal Commission on Mental Illness Report. 1957. London: H.M.S.O.

57. ———. Royal Commission on Medical Education Report 1965-1968. 1968. Cmnd. 3569. London: H.M.S.O.

58. ———. Royal Commission on Local Government Reform in England. 1969. Comnd. 4039. London: H.M.S.O.

59. ———. Secretary of State for Social Services. 1972. National health service reorganization: England. Cmnd. 5055. London: H.M.S.O.

60. ———. Sub-Committee on Child Welfare Centres Report. 1967. London: H.M.S.O.

61. Hill, H. 1971. The Richmond Fellowship, report for the year ending 1971. London: Green and Co.

62. Hill, Sir Denis. 1968. Introduction to The treatment of mental disorders in the community. Daniels and Freeman, eds. London: Bailliere, Tindall and Cassell.

63. ———. 1969. Psychiatric education during a period of social change. Brit. med. J. 1: 205-209.

64. Hobman, D. 1969. A guide to voluntary service. London: H.M.S.O.

65. Hoenig, J. and Crotty, I. 1959. Psychiatric inpatients in general hospitals. Lancet 2: 122.

66. Howells, J. G. 1968. Theory and practice of family psychiatry. Edinburgh: Oliver and Boyd.

67. ———. 1971. Royal college of psychiatrists, special report of the society of clinical psychiatrists. London: The Society of Clinical Psychiatrists.

68. ———. 1972. Family psychiatry for child psychiatrists. London: The Society of Clinical Psychiatrists.

69. ———. (in press). Principles of family psychiatry. New York: Brunner/Mazel.

70. Howells, J. G. and Lickorish, J. R. 1967. Family relations indicator. New York: Brunner/Mazel.

71. Jones, M. 1953. The therapeutic community: a new treatment method in psychiatry. New York: Basic Books.

72. Judson, H. F. 1973. A reporter at large: the British and heroin, Parts I and II. The New Yorker, September 24, pp. 76-113; October 1, pp. 70-112.

73. Kahn, J. H. 1968. The evolution of a community mental health service in a London borough. Mental Hygiene 52: 60-75.

74. Kotulak, R. 1973. London hospital offers life to dying. Detroit Free Press, September 18, Section C., p. 12.
Lancet 1: 543.

75. Krietman, N. 1967. Psychiatric training: a transatlantic viewpoint. Int. J. Psychiat. 4: 451-452.

76. Lawless, J. 1971. The role of the medical profession as an élite. Lancet 1; 543.

77. Lewis, E., Jr. 1973. A heroin maintenance program in the United States. JAMA 223: 539-545.

78. Little, J. C., chmn. 1972. Medical administration in psychiatry. J. G. Howells, ed. Suffolk: The Society of Clinical Psychiatrists.

79. London Membership and Psychiatrists. 1964. Lancet 1: 1085.

80. Marder, L. 1970. Psychiatric experience with a liberalized therapeutic abortion law. Amer. J. Psych. 126: 1230-1236.

81. May, A. R. 1965. The psychiatric nurse in the community. Nursing Mirror, Vol. 121, December.

82. ———. 1968. Organization and efficiency of mental health services. In The treatment of mental disorders in the community. Daniels and Freeman, eds. London: Bailliere, Tindall and Cassell.

83. Mittler, P. 1968. The mental health services. Fabian Research Series 252. London: Fabian Society, June.

84. ———. 1968. Mental health services in the community. Fabian Occasional Paper 4. London: Fabian Society, July.

85. Monro, A. B. 1969. The status of psychiatry in the national health service. Amer. J. Psychiat. 125: 1223-1226.

86. National Council of Social Service. 1968. The caring community. Ref. No. 709/1. London.

87. NHS, Diagnosis for a cure: An injection of political will. 1973. Sunday Times Weekly Review, May 20, pp. 33-34.

88. Oldham, A. J. 1972. A comprehensive service for psychiatry. Health Trends 4: 22-25.

89. Organization for psychiatry. 1963. Lancet 2: 1113.

90. Platt, L. 1967. Medical science: master or servant? Brit. med. J. 4: 439-444.

91. Rehin, G. F. and Martin, F. M. 1963. Psychiatric services in 1975. London: Organization of Political and Economic Planning (PEP).

92. Room, L. E., chmn. 1971. Camden council of social service, Annual report for the year ending 31st March 1971. London.

93. Rosen, D. 1972. Britain gives a fix to its addicts. National Observer, January 1, pp. 1 and 18.

94. Royal Medico-Psychological Association's Memorandum to the Royal Commission on Medical Education, 1966-68. 1968. Brit. J. Psychiat. 114: 1435-39. (reprint).

95. Royal Medico-Psychological Association Reports on Psychiatric Education: Report on the Questionnaire on Postgraduate Training in Psychiatry. 1968. Brit. J. Psychiat. 114: 1441-45. (reprint).

96. Royal Medico-Psychological Association's Memorandum on the Report of the Royal Commission on Medical Education in reply to a letter from the Chief Medical Officer at the Ministry of Health. 1969. Brit. J. Psychiat. 115: 233-241. (reprint).

97. Royal Medico-Psychological Association Reports on Postgraduate Education: Addendum to the Report on the Questionnaire on Postgraduate Training in Psychiatry. 1969. Brit. J. Psychiat. 115: 487-488. (reprint).

98. Royal Medico-Psychological Association's Second Memorandum on the Report of the Royal Commission on Medical Education. 1969. Brit. J. Psychiat. 115: 483-485. (reprint).

99. Sandifer, M. G., Jr.; Horden, A.; Timbuyr, G. C.; and Green, L. M. 1969. Similarities and differences in patient evaluation by U.S. and U.K. psychiatrists. Amer. J. Psychiat. 126: 206-212.

100. Seager, C. P. 1972. Psychiatry and architecture. J. G. Howells, ed. Suffolk: The Society of Clinical Psychiatrists.

101. Seebohm, F., chmn. Report of the committee on local authority and allied personal social services, 1968-69. Cmnd. 3703. London: H.M.S.O.

102. Silverman, M. 1961. A comprehensive department of psychological medicine. Brit. med. J. 2: 698.

103. ———. 1968. The role of the general hospital in psychiatric care. Acta Hospitalia 8: 271-286.

104. Smith, S. 1961. Psychiatry in general hospitals. Lancet 1: 1158.

105. Tetlow, C. 1973. Neglected aspects of psychiatric education. London: Society of Clinical Psychiatrists.

106. Tooth, G. C. and Brooke, E. 1961. Trends in the mental hospital population and their effect on future planning. Lancet 1: 710-713.

107. Training in psychiatry. 1969. Brit. med. J. 1: 394-395.

108. Wallace, J. chmn. 1972. St. Christopher's Hospice. Annual report 1971-1972. Sydenham, England.

109. Walter, G. S. 1970. Psychological and emotional consequences of elective abortion. Obstet.-Gyn. 36: 482-491.

110. Walton, H. J. 1970. The psychiatric component in general practice. Lancet 1: 35-37.

111. Weeks, K. 1966. Psychiatric nurses in the community. Nursing Times 62: 257-258.

112. Wilcher, L. C., chmn. Littlemore Group of Hospitals. 1962. Ninth report of the management committee. London.

113. Wing. J. K. 1966. Evaluating community care of schizophrenic patients in the United Kingdom. In Community Psychiatry. Leigh M. Roberts, ed. Madison: The University of Wisconsin Press.

114. Wing, J. K.; O'Connor, N.; and Lotter, V. 1967. Autistic conditions in early childhood: a survey in Middlesex. Brit. med. J. 3: 389-392.

115. Wing, L.; Wing, J. K.; and Hailey, A. 1968. Camberwell psychiatric case register: third report. 31.12 1964-30.6 London.

116. Wing, L.; Wing, J. K.; Hailey, A.; and Taylor, C. 1967. The use of psychiatric services in three urban areas: an international case register study. Social Psychiatry 2: 158-167.

117. Woodmansey, A. C. 1967. Neglected fundamentals in undergraduate psychiatric education. Brit. J. med. Educ. 1: 183-187.

118. ———. 1967. Science and the training of psychiatrists. Brit. J. Psychiat. 113: 1035-1037.

119. ———. 1970. First principles in psychiatric education. Lancet 1: 610-611.

120. Younghusband, E., chmn. 1959. Report of the working party on social workers in the local authority health and welfare services. H.M.S.O.

ADDITIONAL REFERENCES

121. Goldberg, H. L.; DiMascio, A.; and Chaudhary, B. 1970. A clinical evaluation of prolixin enanthate. Psychosomatics. 11: 173-177.

122. Great Britain. Health Ministry. 1973. Discussion paper on child psychiatric services. London. Pp. 1-10.

index

Norman Rosenzweig, M.D., is chairman of the Department of Psychiatry, Sinai Hospital, Detroit; professor of psychiatry, Wayne State University School of Medicine; and associate clinical professor of psychiatry, College of Human Medicine, Michigan State University. He is chairman, Council of International Affairs, American Psychiatric Association.

The book was designed by Don Ross. The typeface for the text is Press Roman based on Stanley Morison's design of Times New Roman in 1931. The display face is Helvetica designed by Max Miedinger in 1956.

The text is printed on Nicolet Natural text paper and the book is bound in Columbia Mills' Fictionette cloth over binders' boards. Manufactured in the United States of America.